Surprise! It's Vegan

By
Frances Star Graham
VEGAN CHEF

Graham, Frances, author
Surprise! It's Vegan

ISBN (paperback): 979-8-9876603-0-0
ISBN (hardcover): 979-8-9876603-2-4
ISBN (epub ebook): 979-8-9876603-1-7 WITH Video Access
ISBN (epub ebook): 979-8-9876603-3-1 no Video Access
ISBN (ebook for Amazon Kindle): 979-8-9876603-5-5 WITH Video Access
ISBN (ebook for Amazon Kindle): 979-8-9876603-4-8 no Video Access

Library of Congress Control Number: 2023905326

Editor: TheVeganWriter.com
Design and Production: EagleLadyPublishing.com
Food Photography: www.nathrocha.com
Video Tutorial Film Production: www.southmountainfilms.com

Published by:
Frances Graham
frances@cheffrancesstar.com
www.surprise-itsvegan.com

What others are saying...

I collaborated with Chef Frances to bring my vision for my first Vegan Food Tasting Event to life and she blew it out of the water. The menu she curated was amazing! The food she made was better than several vegan food restaurants that I've been to. She is talented, creative, and fun. I would definitely hire Chef Frances again and refer her to my friends and family.
~ *Jennifer*

Frances is absolutely amazing with everything she prepares. I have used her several times for business events and every time we all leave very satisfied on all levels—her professionalism, talent with her food creations, as well as hearty tasty portions. Communication is excellent and prices are reasonable.
Thank you, Frances!
~ *Julia with Halo's Holistic Healing Center*

As a non-vegan customer, I can tell you that Frances is not only an amazing and incredibly talented chef but an excellent resource for explaining the benefits of plant-based eating. She truly cares about people and their health and spends time answering any questions you might have. Her professionalism makes you feel like your event is in perfect hands.
~ *Nicole*

Frances cooked for an event, and it was vegan. All I can say is heavenly! Everything was delicious, tasty and filling. I will definitely use her for some of my events for sure.
~ *Doretta with Ladies Leaving Legacies, LLC.*

Her food is so delicious! I had the Caesar Pasta Salad with Baby Kale. It was so full of flavor and filling. I loved it. Her zucchini bread was delicious as well; such a great way to get more greens in your diet wrapped in a sweet treat (but not too sweet, just right). Yum!
~ *Crystal*

Frances taught us how to create her Winter Power Bowl; it was AMAZING! I can't wait to share her food and talents with everyone I know. Thank you.
~ *Nicole with The Party Porter*

I attended a cooking class/demonstration with Frances and it was phenomenal! The meals she/we made were absolutely delicious and she is very knowledgeable about all the ingredients she uses. I could tell she really loves what she does, and I can't wait to try more of her creations.
~ *Mallory*

Featured on Cover

Cauliflower Power Side Salad with Agave Mustard Dressing

Recipe on Page 45

Dedication

This book is dedicated to all my persistent customers. Thank you for encouraging me to share my recipes in the form of a book. I have much gratitude for you kindly pushing me to share my cooking secrets with you.

Contents

Acknowledgments

Many thanks to my husband, Larry, for always supporting my culinary business and any of my passions. To my children, Maraya and Cameron, for having such a positive attitude while I used you as my little guinea pigs to try my food.

Additional thanks go directly to my mom, Kathy, for being the best cook and plant person for our big family growing up. To my mother-in-law, Dawn, for being the absolute best mentor to me as a master baker of baked goodies. To Bonnie, an amazing cook and mentor, for soul and comfort food, and for helping me season my food to nourish others.

I am grateful beyond measure for the opportunity to attend culinary school. I will never forget all the chefs and chef instructors who spent countless hours mentoring me in the culinary field.

Julia, thank you for supporting my culinary business by hosting many food events at your holistic healing center in Mesa, Arizona. It's been a fun ride.

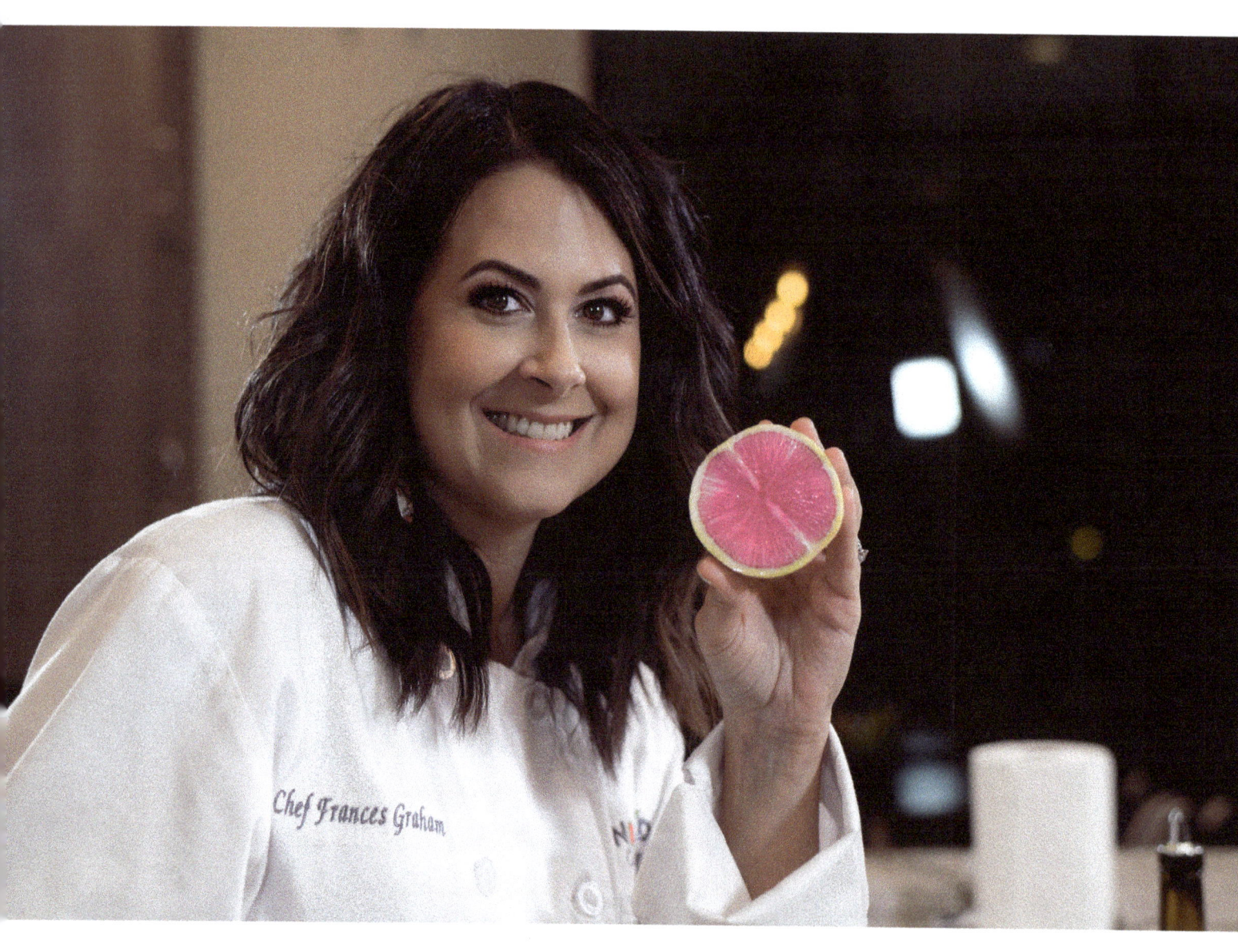

Introduction

Growing up in the Midwest in the small city of Springfield, Illinois was a life experience that may be familiar to many. I had the privilege of growing up with many trees around me. They served as a canopy of the perfect shelter for me during childhood and most of my twenties. I was always connected to them in a way that still seems natural yet necessary to my identity. Not until I moved to the desert at the age of thirty-three did I appreciate the energy and value of those massive trees. My soulful true-self home away from home.

At the age of three, I would play in the soil for hours making mud pies in my rugged monster tire sandbox. I was so proud of my carefully crafted mud pies. Presently, I work as a private vegan chef, where I genuinely develop dishes and recipes, which is a creative outlet and true therapy for my self-worth and healing process.

A big part of my recipe creation is sharing these tasty dishes with others. Since I was 17, I have worked in many restaurants as a hostess, waitress, bartender, bar manager, food expediter, and food prep worker, and I attended culinary school in Dallas, Texas. I went on to work with many famous chefs at fundraisers and events. However, many connections and experiences pushed me to work in the culinary field as my chosen career later in life. I did not start my culinary business until I was 42 years old, and now at age 46, I am so grateful to have

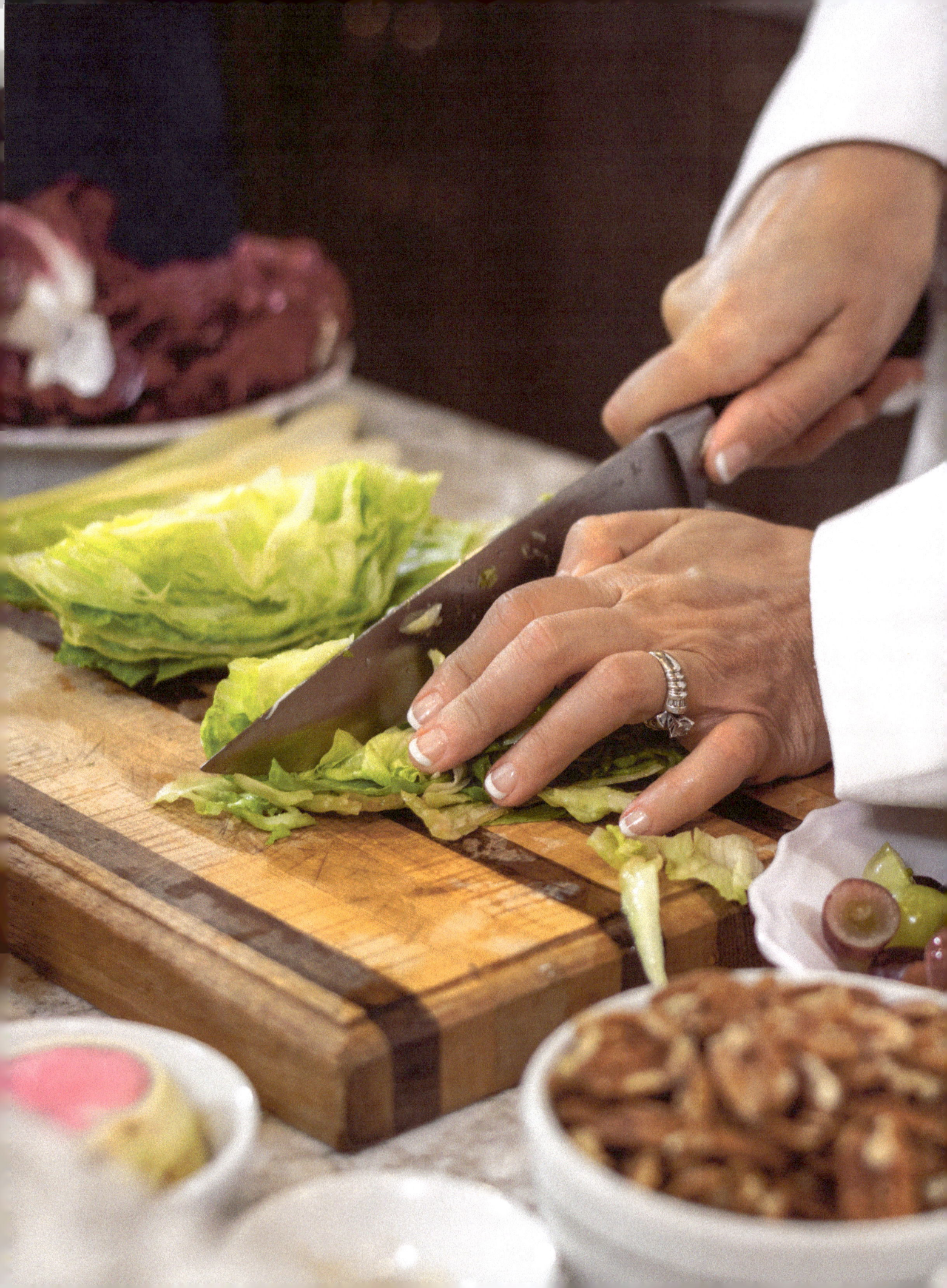

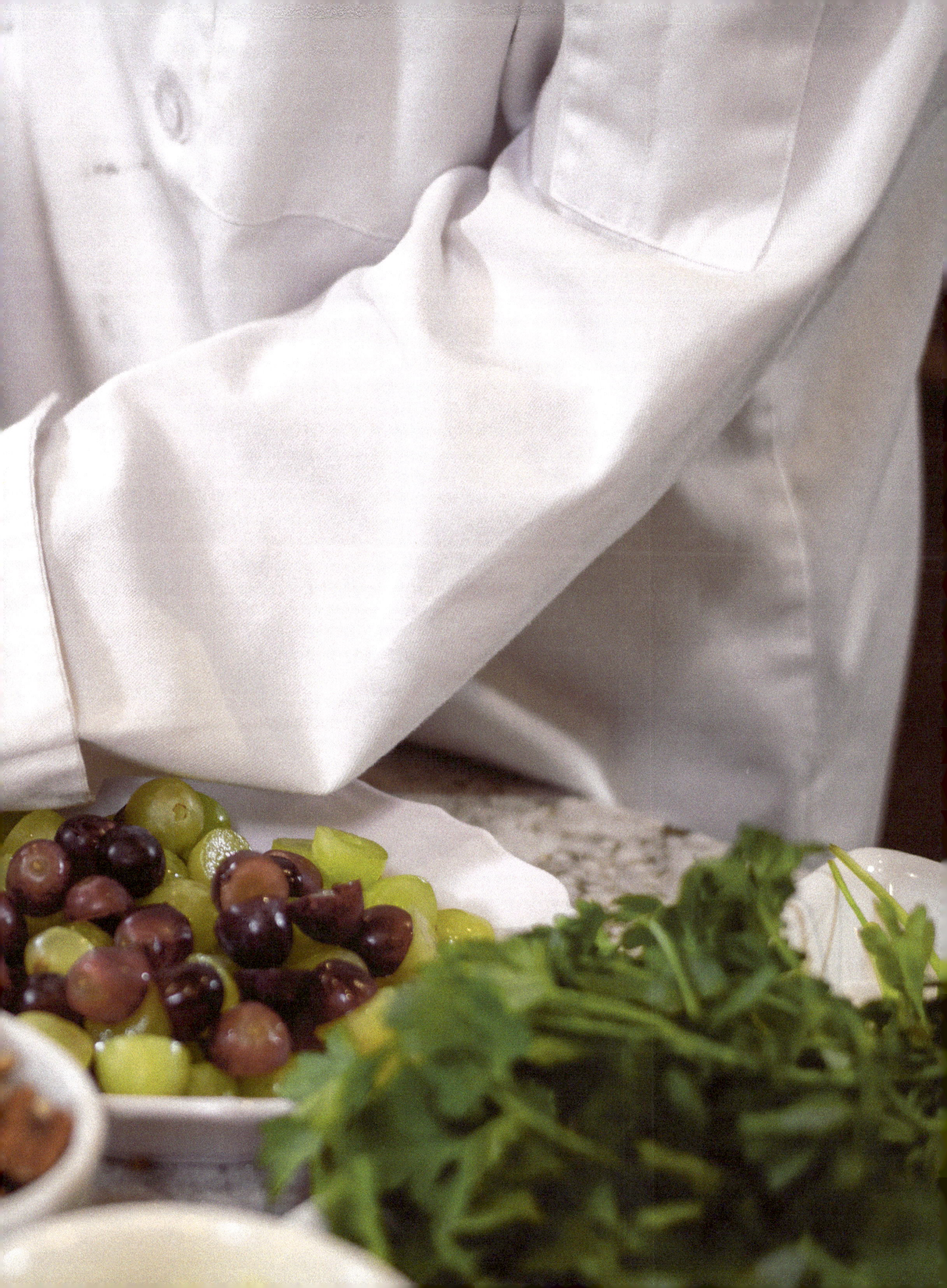

created this cookbook for you with chef-inspired recipes of vegan comfort food.

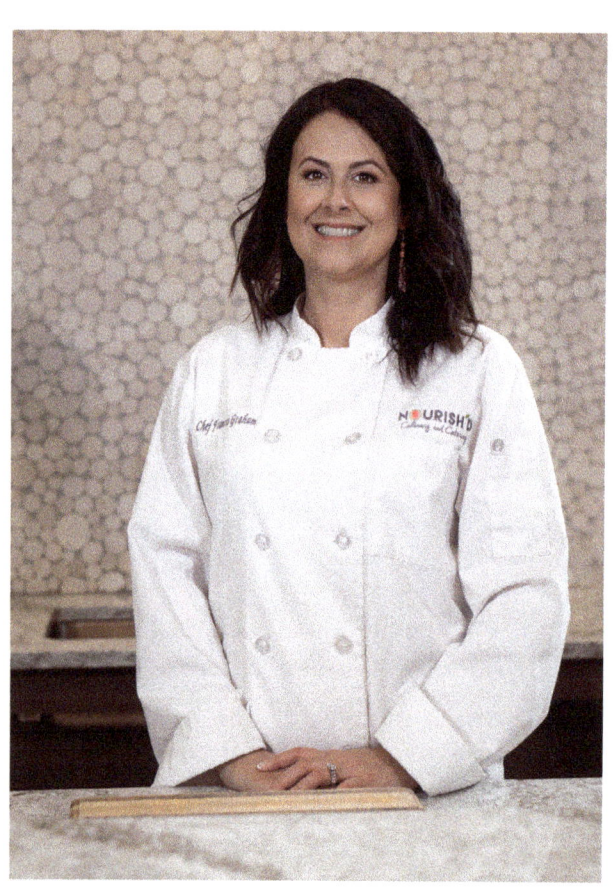

I will never forget one of my most raw childhood memories of my mother's vegetable garden. The vegetable garden started every spring and ended around mid-October. The garden's permanent home was in the backyard of a red shack and make-shift house where our family lived. I was the oldest of three children already born at that time. My two younger brothers loved to follow me around like puppy dogs waiting to see what imaginative game I would make up for us to play together.

Living off our rented land was the reality of our survival. Our family was poor and hard-working. This land we inhabited was a prized and precious commodity. The rewarding result was a half-acre garden my mother thoughtfully planned, planted, and nurtured. She taught me to weed and dig around the green goddess-type collards and cabbages. My little hands would bleed and throb with joy at the chance to pull up any vegetation from the ground.

I remember chasing rabbits out of the garden and past the wire and wood fence next to the railroad tracks. I wanted to make sure they did not eat our prized jumbo carrots and radishes. My connection to the garden and its produce was such a cherished and clear memory

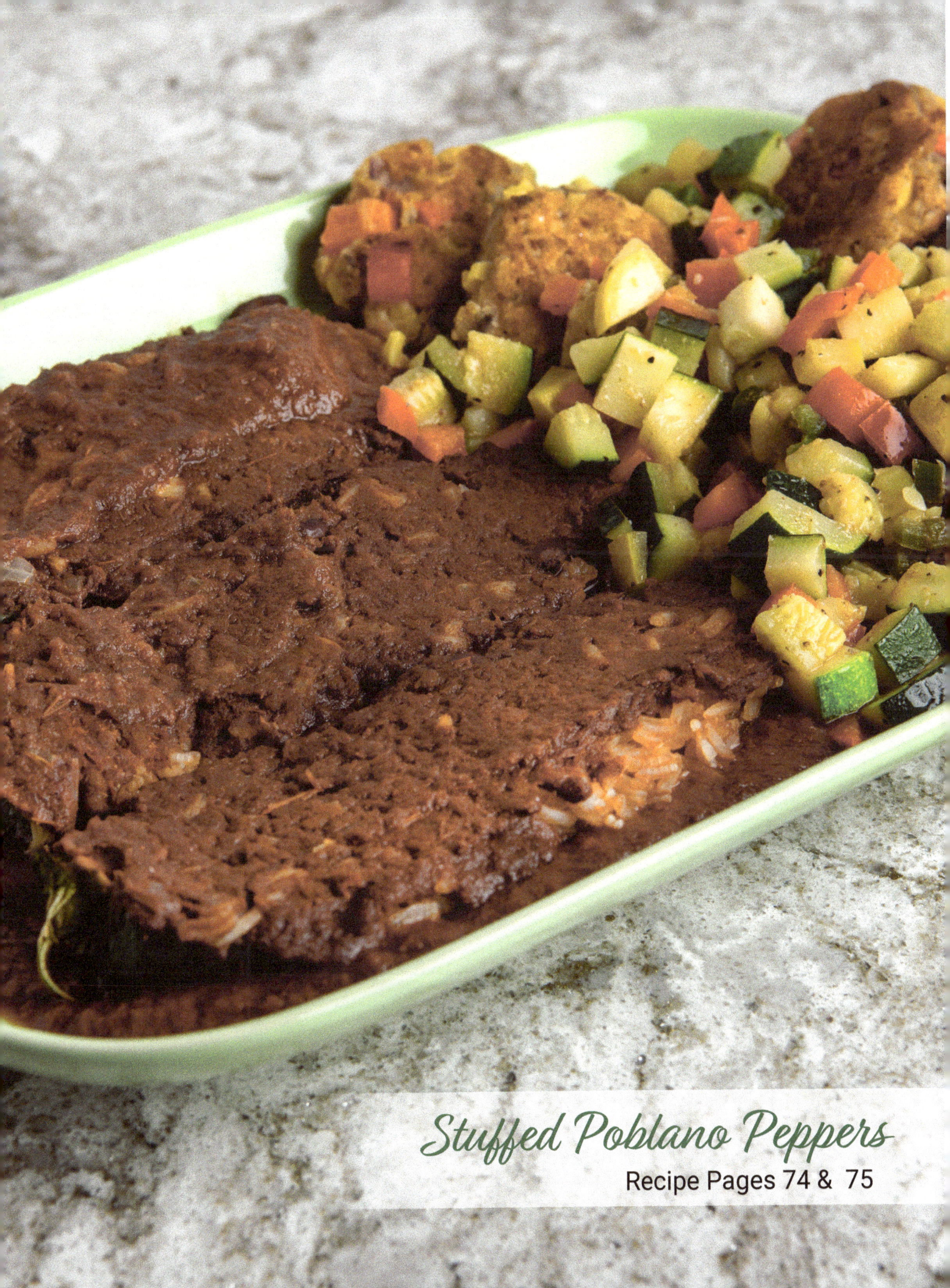

Stuffed Poblano Peppers
Recipe Pages 74 & 75

of my good and bad relationship with food. Can you remember your first connection with food or fresh produce? I think it's crucially important to the rest of our lives and how we eat and thrive throughout our lifetime.

We share similar experiences as humans that form and shape who we are to the core. Years and years went by before I realized I wasn't being my authentic self. Through the years, I spent too much time indoors, worked for corporate America, ate processed foods 24/7, and ignored my horrible digestive issues for decades. I was on the oh-so-popular train of always focusing on being an overachiever in life without taking care of myself. Ignoring my self-care created a lack of energy and vibrance I very much needed.

I had many pleasant and rewarding life lessons throughout my lifetime that I am proud to have experienced. On the other side of things, I did ignore the years of trauma from ages 5 to 23, which festered in my body like a major time bomb. By the time I was 29, I had a bleeding ulcer and many years of fatigue and bedridden days ahead of me.

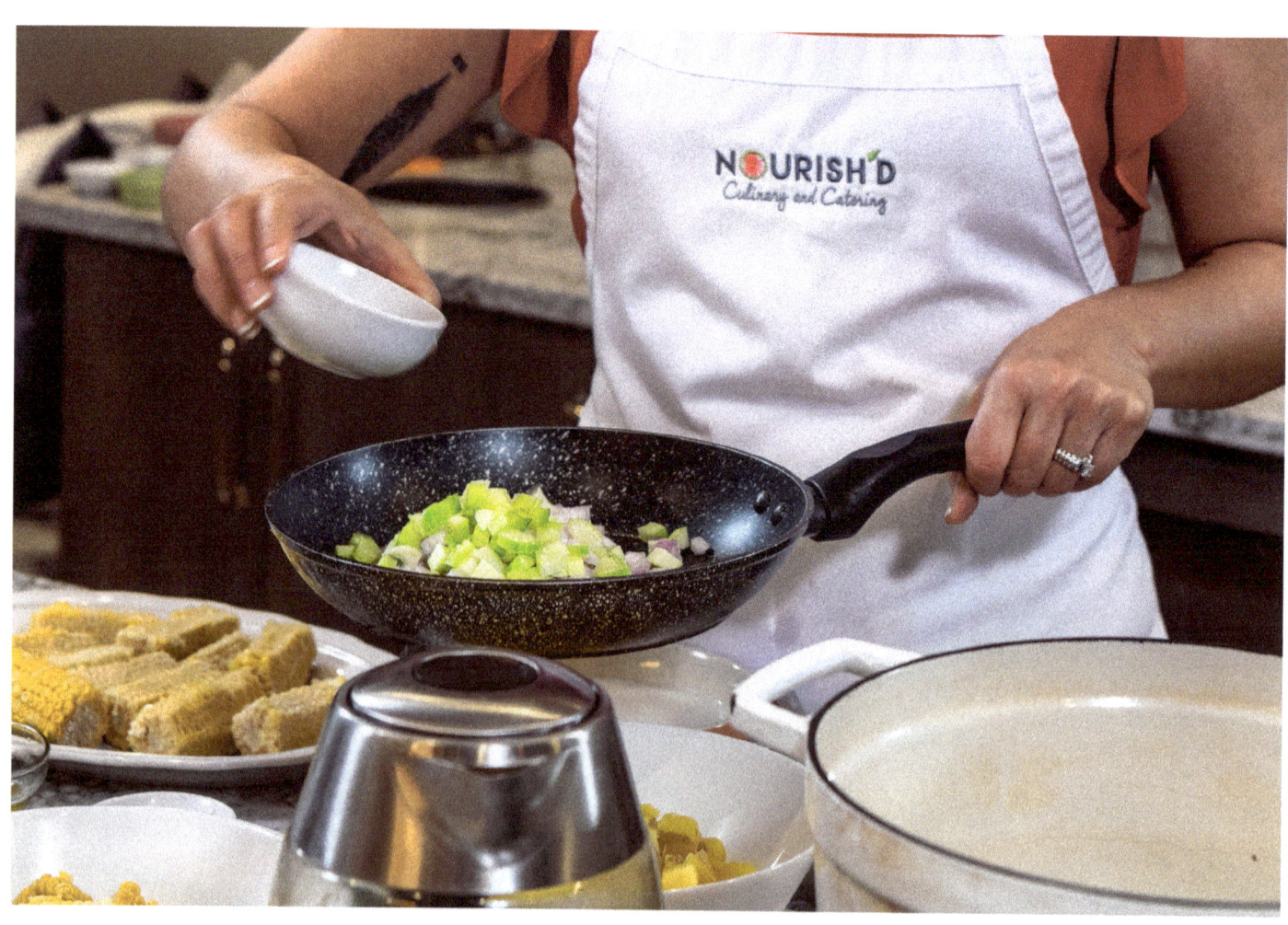

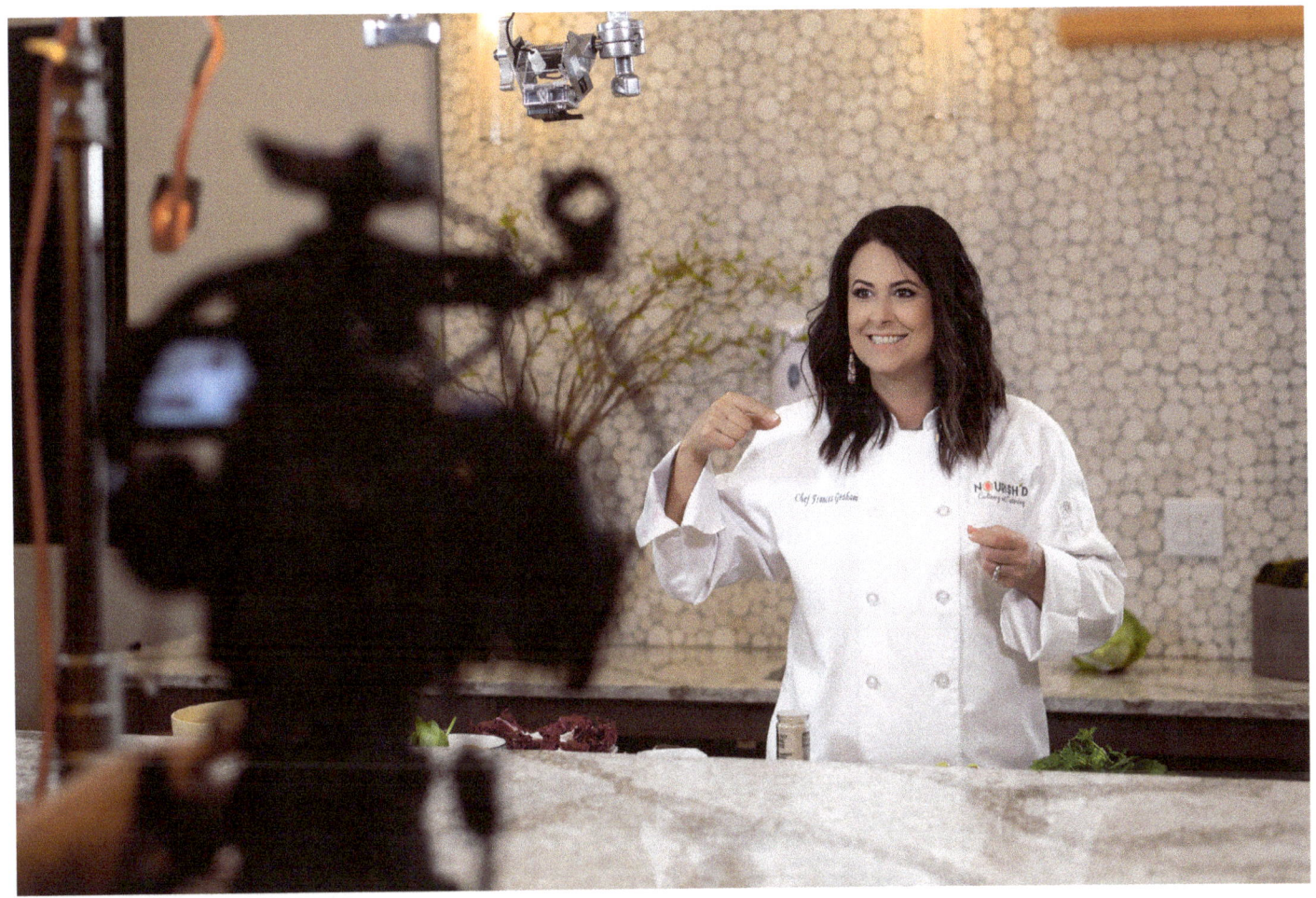

Age 33 was a defining moment: I was diagnosed with Hashimoto's Thyroid Disease. Weight gain, fatigue, heart issues, and chronic pain were making me miserable daily. I also had given birth to a daughter and son, but barely stayed alive during my pregnancies since I wasn't diagnosed and therefore not treated for this thyroid condition until well after they were born. I still had no idea that diet and fitness were the areas of my life that I needed to get back on track to live a meaningful life without sickness.

In 2013, at the age of 36, I was diagnosed with Sjögren's Systemic Autoimmune Disease and Crest Syndrome (a form of Scleroderma). Sjögren's is an immune system disorder characterized by dry eyes and mouth. With this disorder, my body's immune system attacks its own healthy cells that produce saliva and tears. Crest is a chronic hardening and tightening of the skin and connective tissues in the body. The combination of Hashimoto's, Sjögren's, and Crest greatly affected my lifestyle when it came to working a 9-to-5 job, raising my family, and functioning as a healthy woman in general.

One day at end of 2013, my heart

stopped, and I lost consciousness for a few minutes while going through a routine bladder test at an in-patient doctor's appointment. I was left alone in the room and fell to the floor after passing out. Fortunately, the doctors and nurses were able to revive me after working on me for a good 20 minutes. I couldn't hear or speak to anyone for an hour after this happened. I found out later that I had another condition that caused me to lose my electrolytes too quickly. As I was walking to my car after that appointment, I started to feel weird new energy around me. My life was getting ready to change. I was sick and tired of being defenseless. I needed to be healthy, and I had no idea where to start.

Eating differently was the beginning of my life change, but it didn't happen overnight. For three years, I researched how to change my diet. Intuitively, I knew that, for me, change needed to be gradual. I had so many challenges ahead of me. Growing up in the Midwest, we had a diet that was overly focused on using meat, dairy, and eggs in our meals and even in most of our snacks. Our Midwest, American diet was rich and did not have much green stuff with the vitamins and minerals that our bodies need, which was especially challenging for my anemic body.

In 2015, I decided to begin a three-year process of changing to a vegan lifestyle. I wanted this change to be permanent, not a fad. Every three months, I cut out one type of animal product: one quarter, no more beef; one quarter, no more pork; one quarter, no more poultry; one quarter, no more dairy. The last two years of transitioning consisted of a pescatarian eating style. Pescatarians do not eat meat but do eat fish.

January 2018 was when I fully and permanently became vegan, and I did not look back. Being vegan was a life change that greatly improved my health. The combination of the new diet and exercise (qigong is my energy practice) put me in remission. What did that mean for my life and health? It means that I no longer have to endure extreme symptoms from the diseases I was medically diagnosed with,

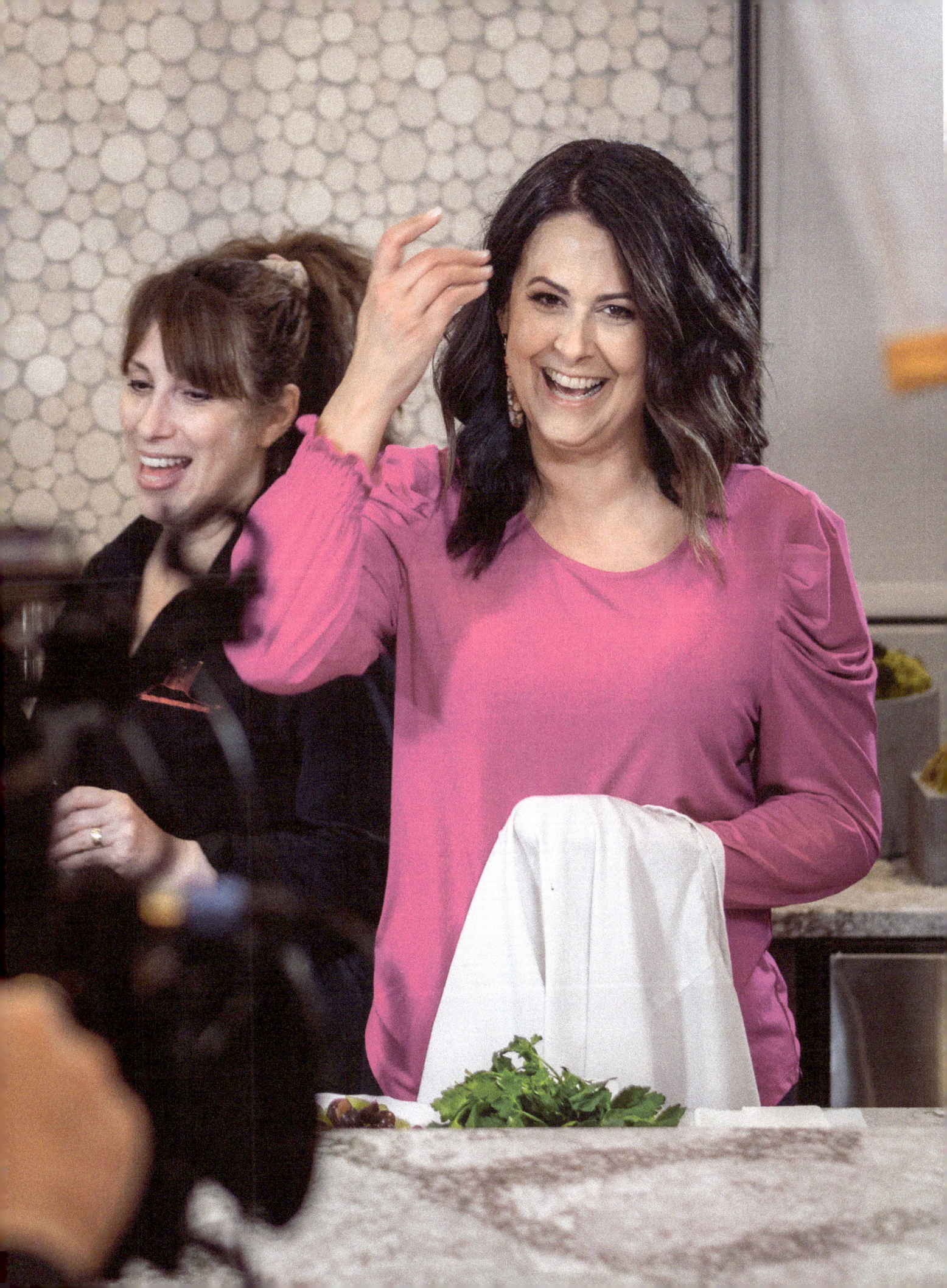

and I regenerated my thyroid gland to its normal size.

In 2010, I was told that the Hashimoto's was so severe that 40 percent of my thyroid gland was missing, and I was in a hypothyroid state. That's right! I regenerated my thyroid gland. A medical miracle the doctors could not explain after seeing these amazing results during a brain and throat MRI. I knew exactly what healed me: the nourishing, alkaline, and anti-inflammatory plants I was consuming daily.

After a long and exhausting journey with these diseases, I immersed myself in creating fun and new plant recipes for the masses. With increased energy, I took advantage of the eight months of mostly pleasant weather in Arizona—where I have lived since 2010—and started hiking all over this beautiful state. I had the pleasure of hosting many cooking classes, events, and community gatherings where I introduced people to tasty and rewarding healthy foods they could make for themselves and their loved ones. I was

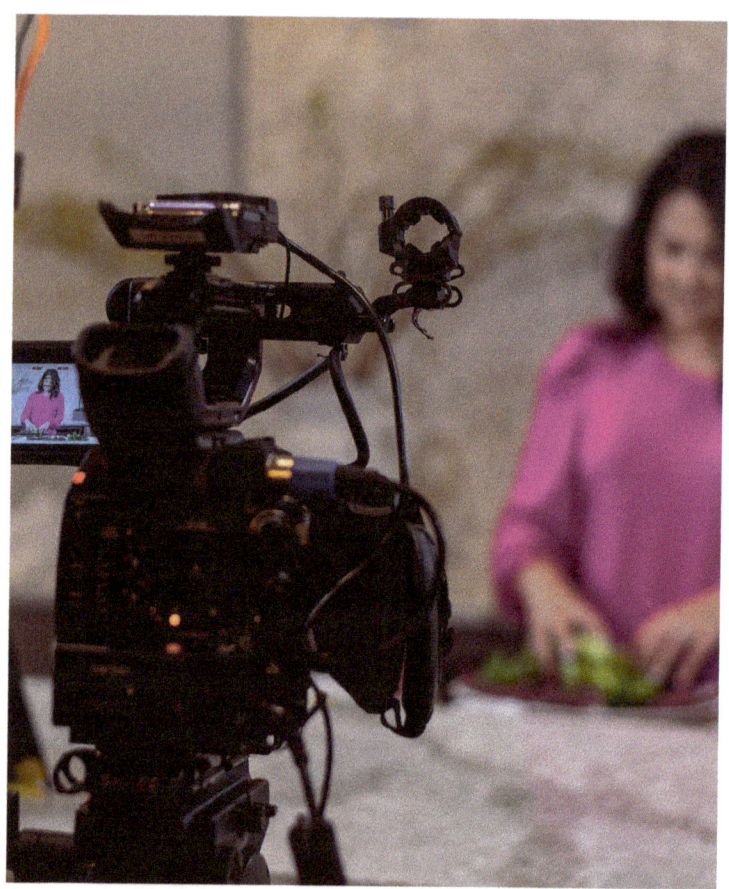

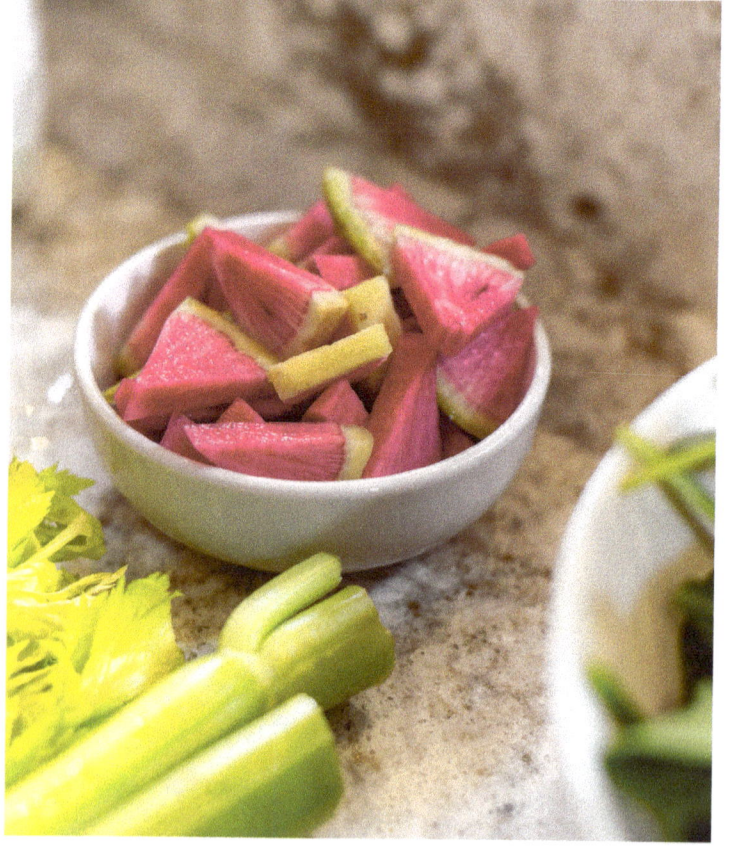

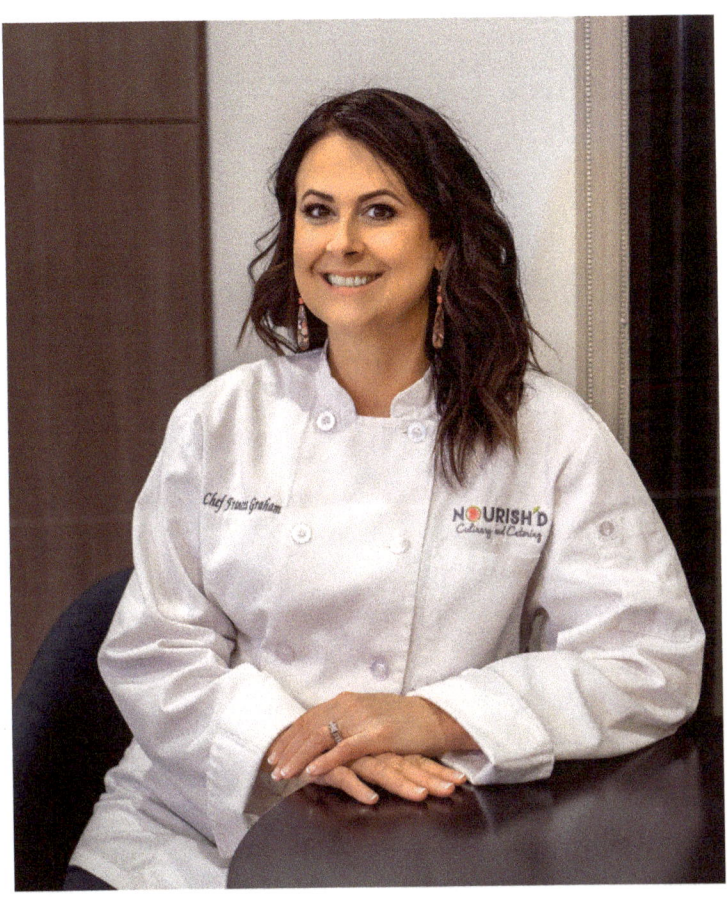

lucky enough to be a private chef for meat eaters, always surprising them with filling, comforting food. They would often say, "We didn't miss the meat at all!" and "That cheese tasted so close to the real thing!"

Through the years, this positive feedback from my customers and friends inspired me to write my first cookbook. I am overjoyed to introduce you to Surprise! It's Vegan. In this cookbook, I do not highlight too many faux meat dishes, but rather showcase the unique flavor and versatility of many vegetables and a few fruits, along with cultural comfort food dishes. As a chef, I take my foundational training and restaurant experience to a whole new level with the details I share with you about each recipe.

You could take a few of these recipes and create a menu to open a plant-based restaurant or host a gathering where you introduce vegan dishes to meat eaters. I will admit that many recipes lean toward the Mediterranean diet, and many are remakes of classic dishes. I created sauces

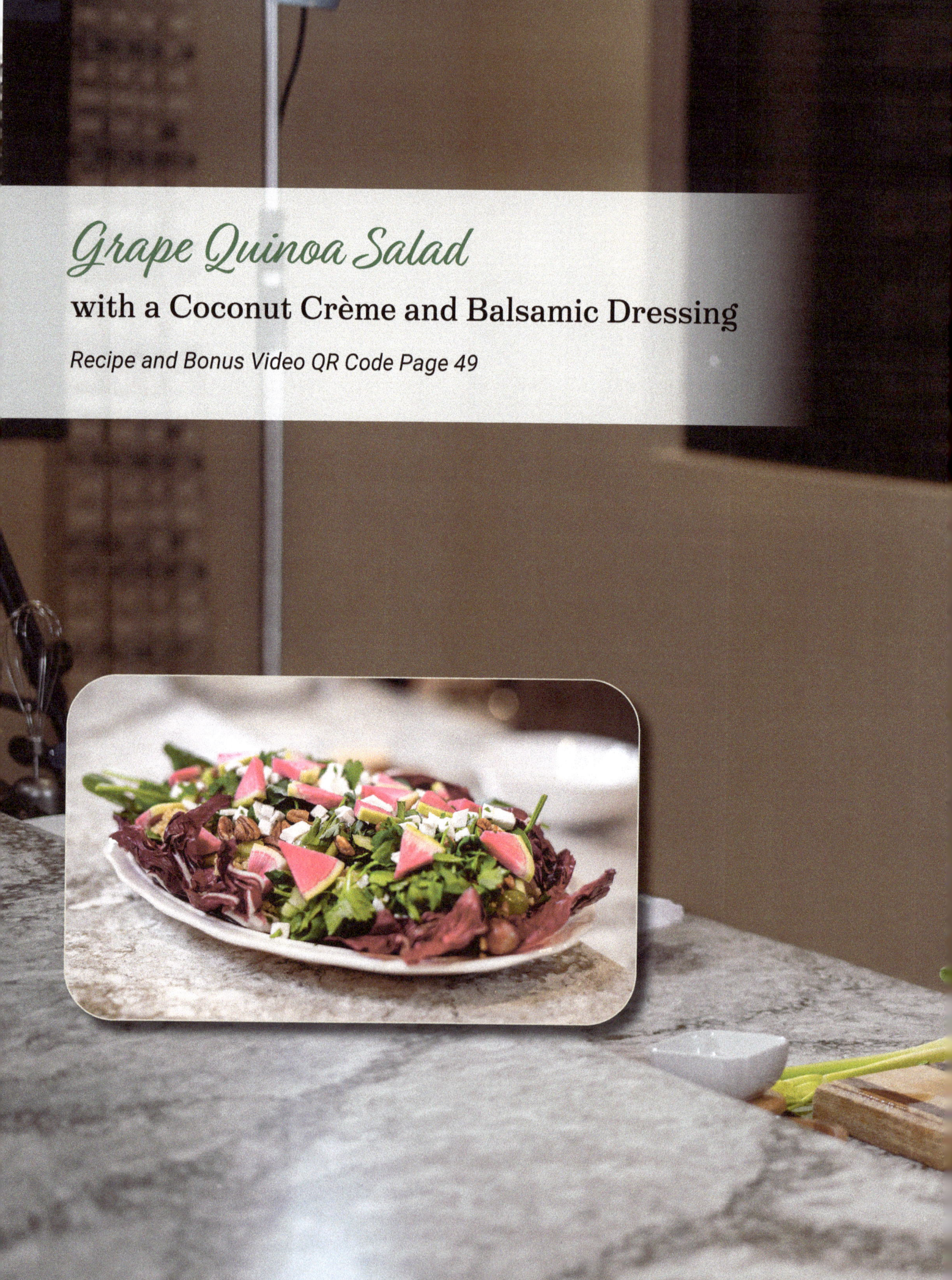

Grape Quinoa Salad

with a Coconut Crème and Balsamic Dressing

Recipe and Bonus Video QR Code Page 49

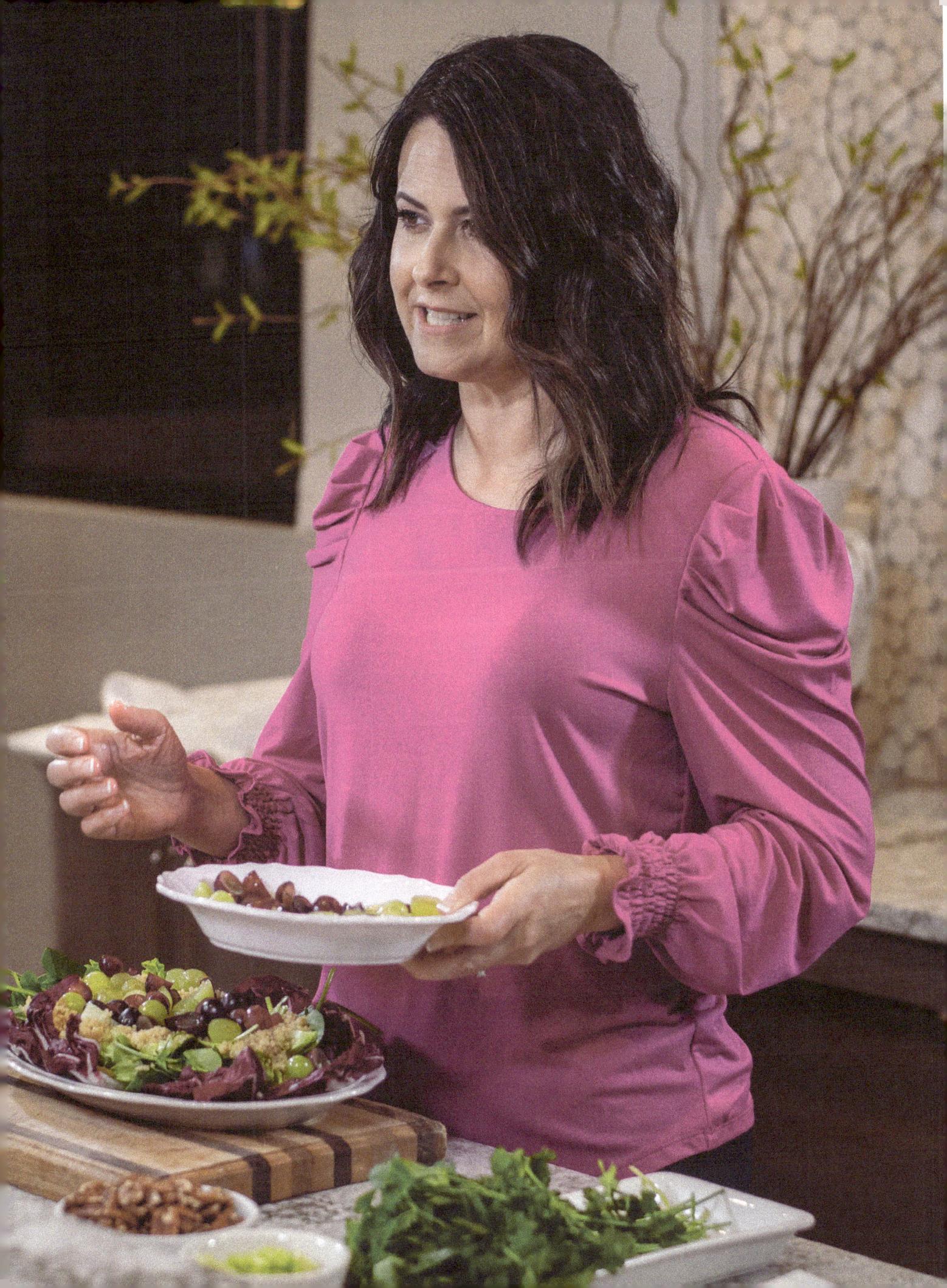

and dressings that you will not see anywhere else.

Many of the vegetable dishes are alkaline, meaning that they are not acidic and therefore are the healthiest for your body systems. Although I have nutritional training, I'm not claiming to provide medical or certified nutritional advice, especially in any type of clinical sense. The recipes all have a gluten-free option available, and many recipes are gluten-free already. Healthy oils, low-sugar, and no-sugar options are used frequently.

After working with hundreds of people to help them get healthy through energy practice and diet changes, I'm confident what I share will benefit you and your health. Take the pressure off your diet goals by not changing your diet overnight. Instead, try these chef-inspired recipes and have fun with the new textures and flavors. You will be surprised at how close to the meat-based counterparts these dishes taste. Also, you will feel pure satisfaction when your tummy is full without all the low-energy crashes after meals.

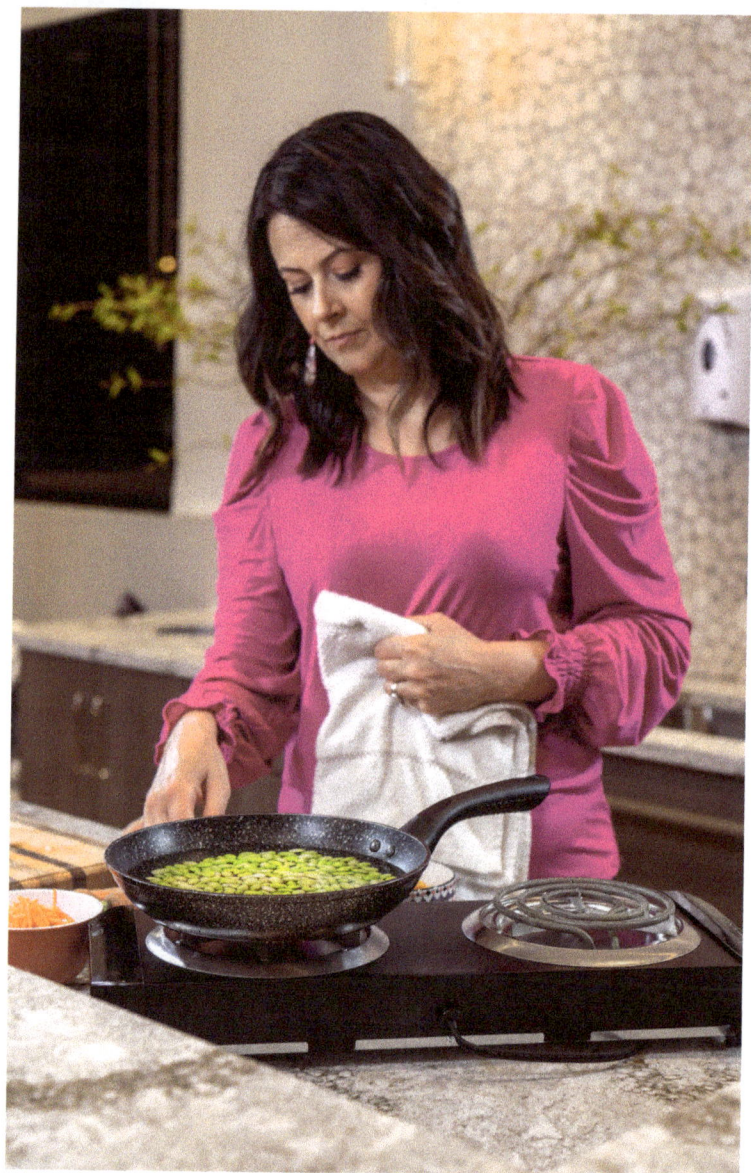

Comfort food is all about the emotional state your whole body is in after consuming a meal or attending a family event that has great food. You can also serve these dishes at a party and you're sure to be the most impressive cook as a host or a contributing guest. Folks will be asking you to share your recipe and others will want you to make their favorites again.

Thank you for reading this cookbook; I assure you that it's not your typical cookbook. You will find video recipes by scanning the QR code on some pages, along with a thumbnail photo of the recipe. Scan the code with your phone and watch the video from anywhere. My goal with this cookbook is to ensure it doesn't merely sit on a shelf unused; I'm confident you will pick it up time and time again, making old favorites and discovering new ones.

There are 44 recipes, which should not overwhelm those new to cooking, but seasoned foodies will be delighted with its easy yet descriptive and educational recipes. Each recipe is a chef-created dish that will impress your friends, family, or work colleagues. Enjoy this health-improving adventure—it's not just a cookbook.

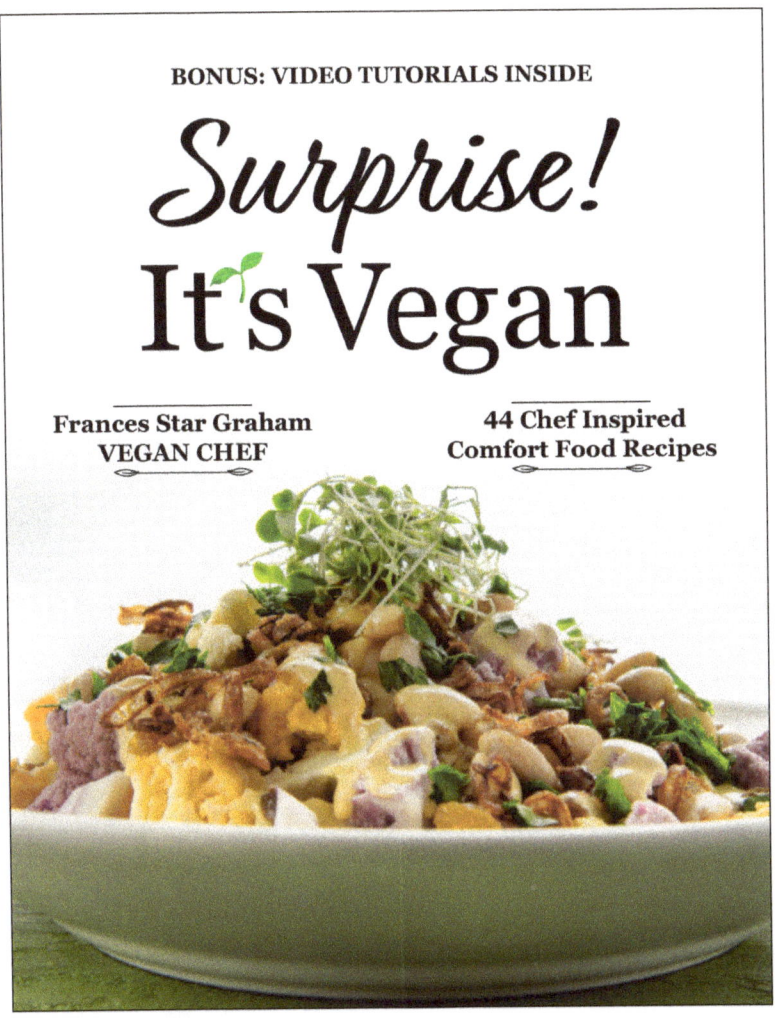

BONUS: VIDEO TUTORIALS INSIDE

Surprise!
It's Vegan

Frances Star Graham
VEGAN CHEF

44 Chef Inspired
Comfort Food Recipes

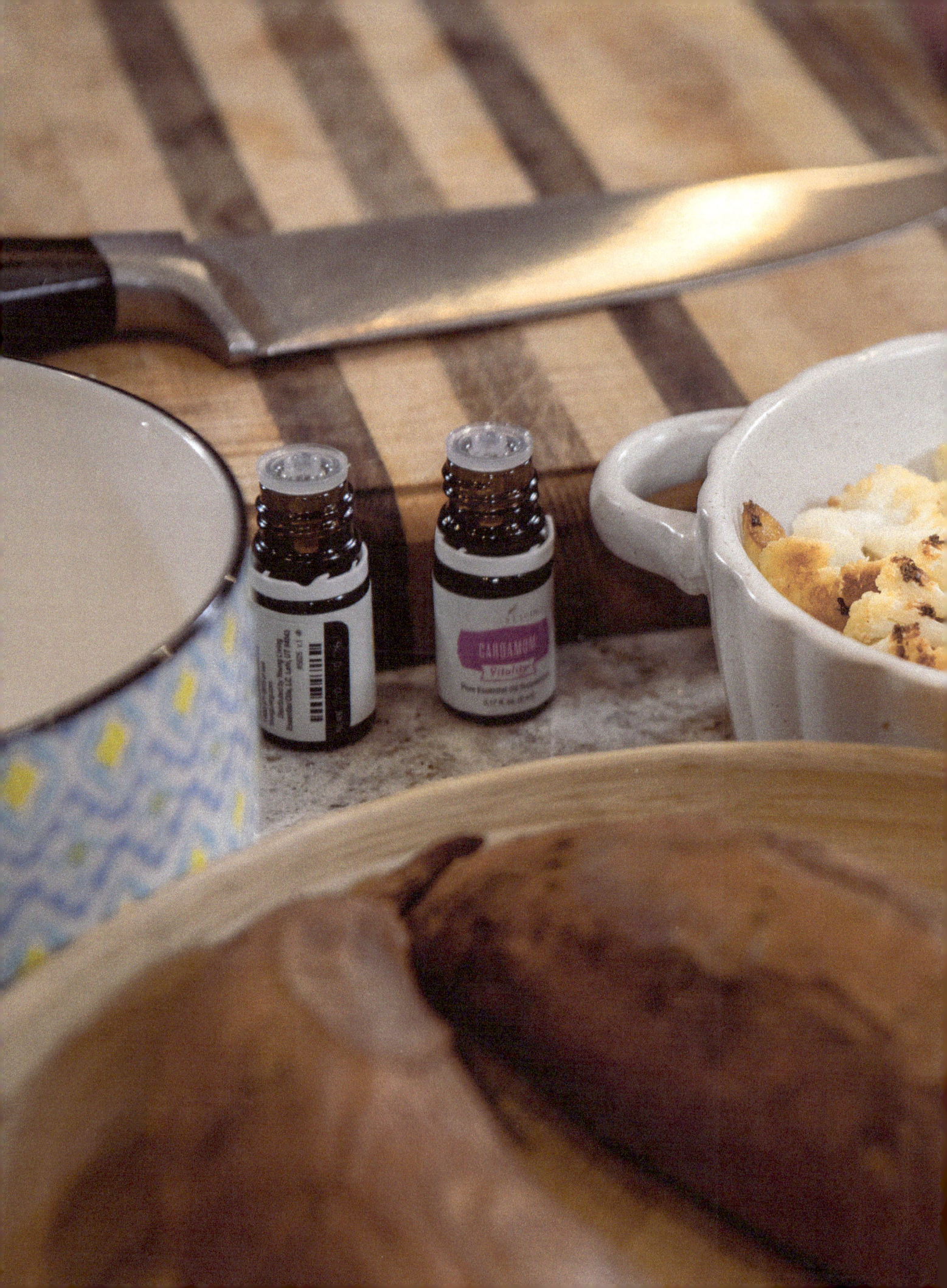

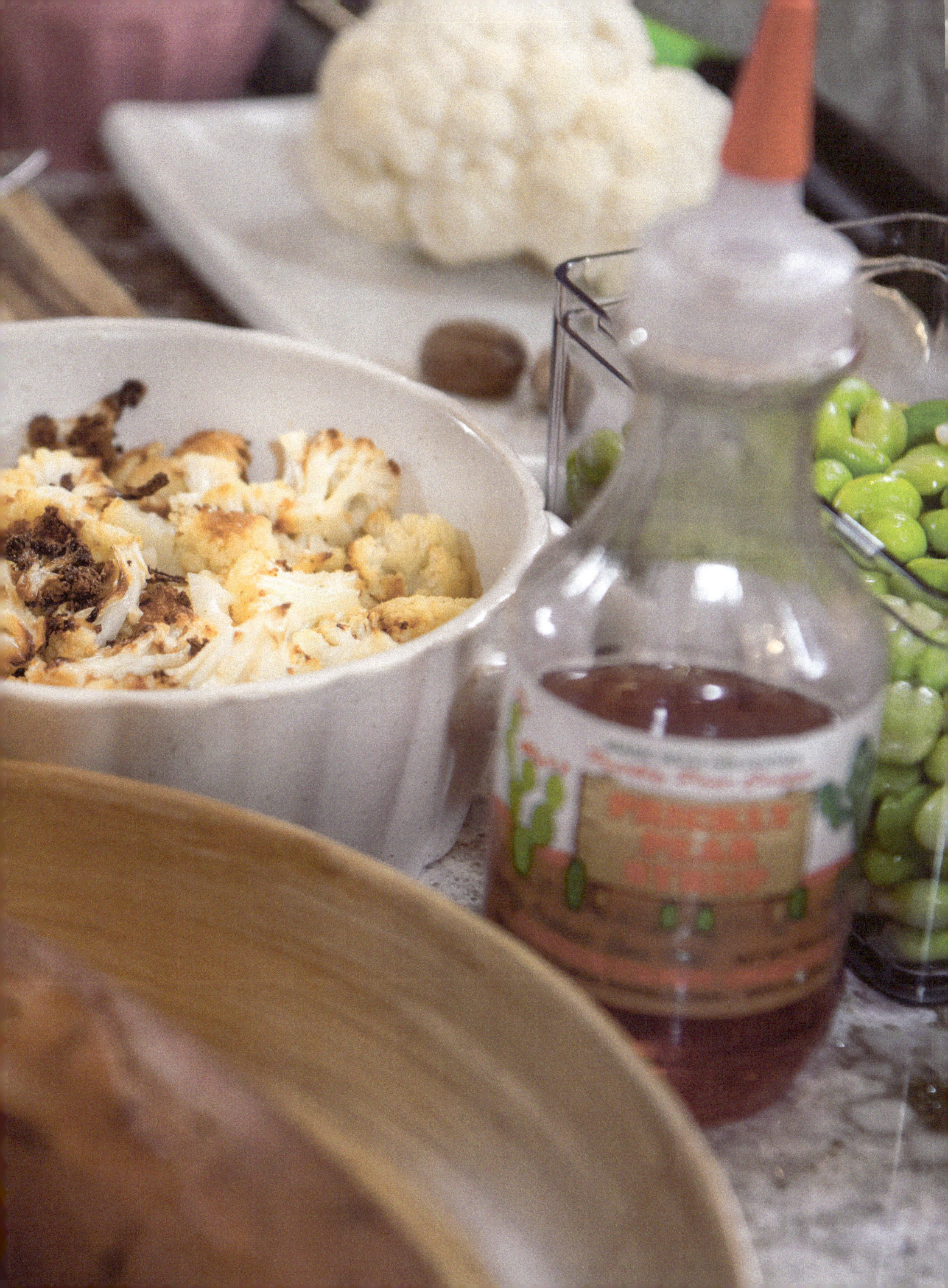

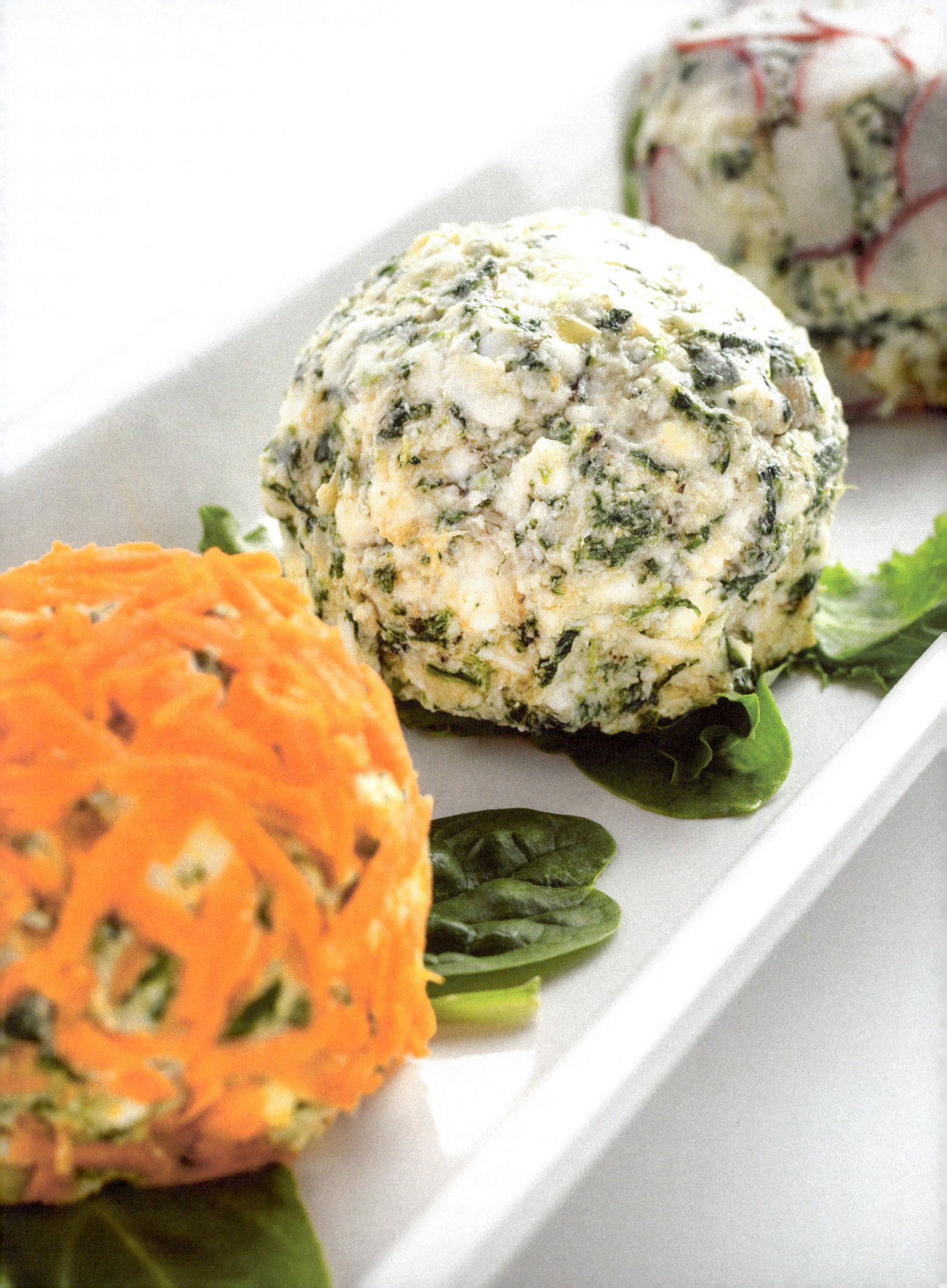

Appetizers and Soups

Vegan Wild Rice Mushroom Soup

Midwest-Style Vegan Corn Chowder

Chef Frances' Famous Feta Cheeseballs

Stuffed Mushrooms with Microgreens

French Onion Soup

Featured Opposite Page:
Chef Frances' Famous Feta Cheeseballs

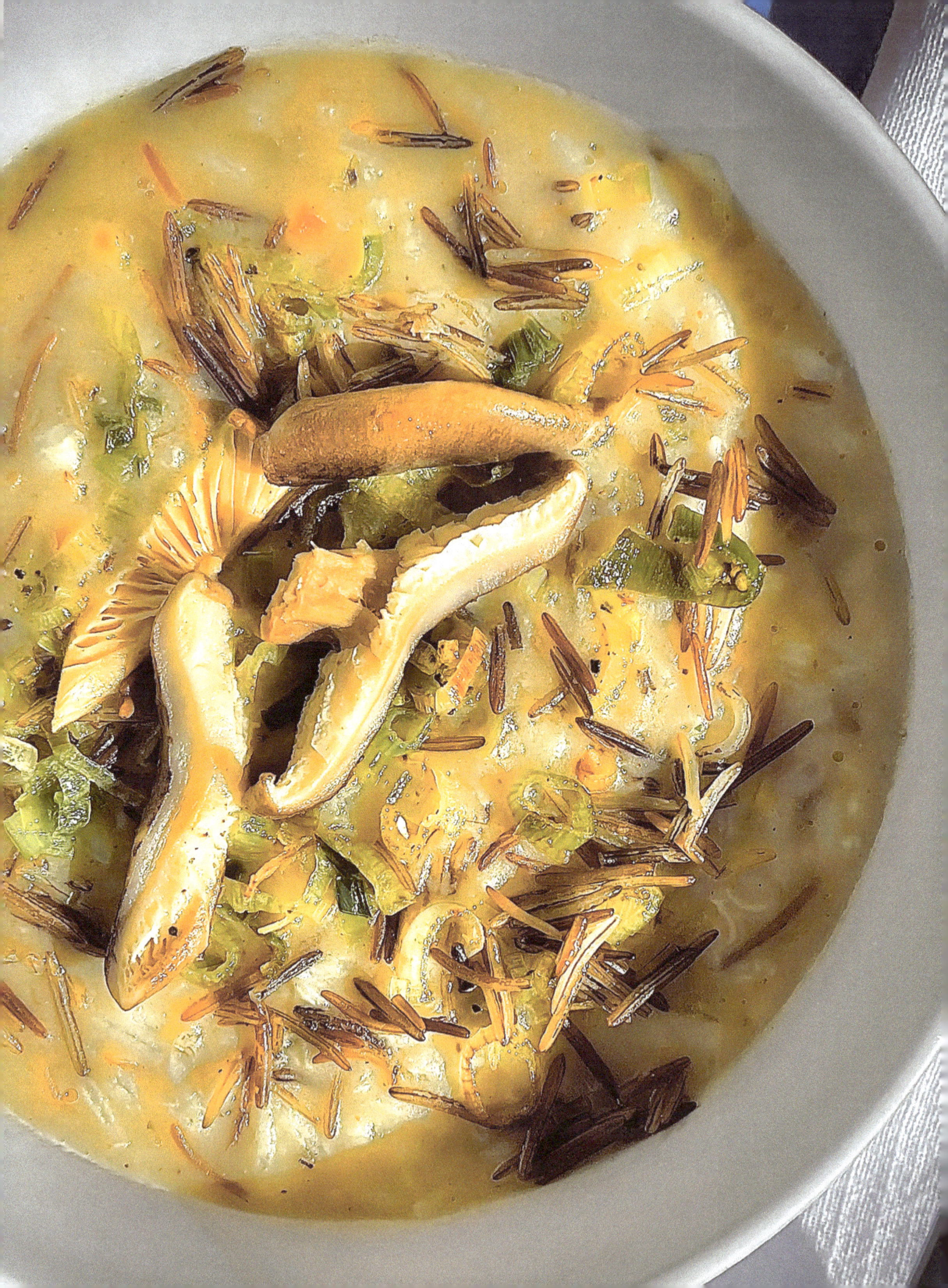

Vegan Wild Rice Mushroom Soup

Equipment: Large Dutch oven or 8 qt. pot, medium pot, chef knife, medium mixing bowl

1 cup of dry black wild rice

2 cups of dry white rice

2 tablespoons of Miyoko's vegan unsalted butter

2 tablespoons of extra virgin olive oil

1 teaspoon of cornstarch

¼ cup of carrots, celery, and onion, finely diced (equaling ¾ cup)

4 cups of miso broth (from a carton)

4 cloves of garlic, finely minced

1½ cups of shiitake mushrooms, rehydrated or fresh

1 leek, thinly sliced

Salt and pepper

½ teaspoon of cayenne pepper

Directions:

Precook both types of rice separately for 10 minutes on a low simmer with tight-fitting lids, using water for the cooking liquid: 2 cups of white rice and 3 cups of water; 1 cup of black rice with 2 cups of water. Cook the black rice first and then the white rice or cook the black rice and at the same time cook the white rice in a rice cooker. It's okay if both varieties are undercooked; they will cook again within the soup.

Empty both rice mixtures into a bowl and set aside. Combine all veggies except mushrooms and the leek in a saucepan with 1 tablespoon of extra virgin olive oil and cook until slightly tender—5 minutes on medium heat. Remove veggies from the saucepan and set aside.

Add vegan butter to a large saucepan and melt on low heat. Turn up the heat and add miso broth slowly while whisking. Add cornstarch and continue whisking. The soup will slightly thicken. Add salt and pepper, cayenne pepper, and any other herbs you would like for your own flavor profile, such as thyme. Add cooked rice, cover, and simmer on low for 5 minutes.

Slice the leek into thin rounds, and fry in the additional tablespoon of olive oil for 5 minutes. Remove from heat with a slotted spoon and set aside for garnish. Add shiitake mushrooms to the same saucepan, additional oil is not needed as there should be some remaining from leeks, and sauté for 3 minutes. Set aside for garnish.

Serve soup in small deep bowls. Garnish with fried leeks and sautéed mushrooms.

Serves 4 to 6.

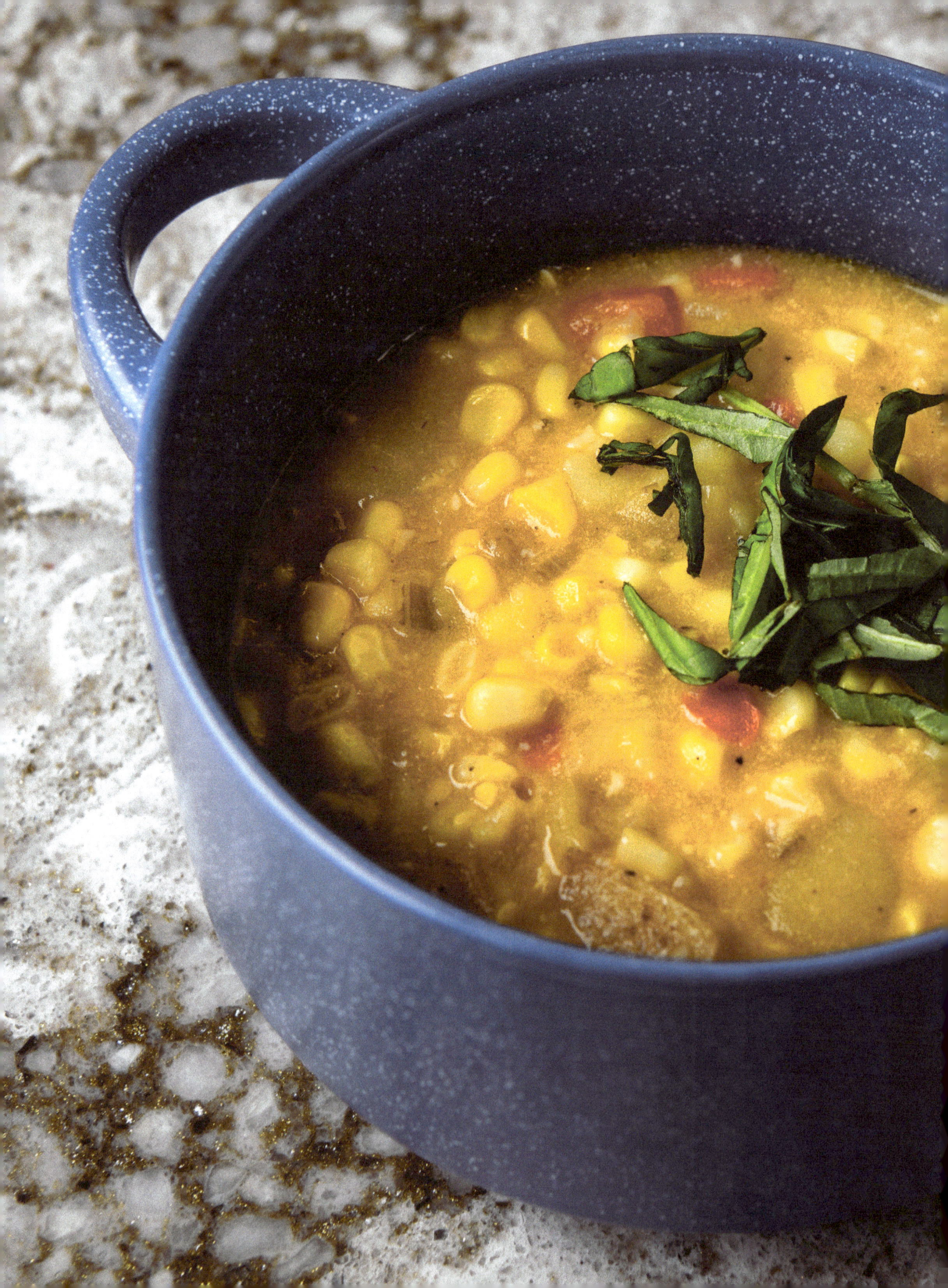

Midwest-Style Vegan Corn Chowder

Equipment: Dutch oven or large, deep soup pan, medium saucepan, sharp serrated knife

6 cobs of sweet corn

4 medium Yukon Gold potatoes

½ cup celery with celery leaves, finely diced

1 red bell pepper, diced

2 shallots, minced

2 cloves of garlic, finely chopped

1 tablespoon of gluten-free flour

2 tablespoons of Miyoko's vegan butter

4 cups of hot vegetable broth

1 can of coconut crème

2 cups of macadamia milk

1 teaspoon of Louisiana Hot Sauce

2 tablespoons of basil, finely minced

Salt and Pepper to taste
   (around 1 teaspoon each or less)

2 bay leaves, dried

Bonus VIDEO TUTORIAL

 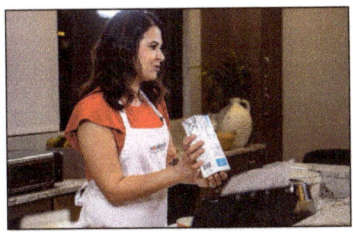

Password: Z1977Fsg1111$
Note: Save the password to your browser
for easier access

Directions:

Boil cobs of corn on medium-high for 7 minutes. Remove and cool. Cut the kernels from the cob with a serrated knife and collect them inside a medium bowl. Save cobs and set aside. Sauté red bell pepper, celery, shallots, and garlic in 1 tablespoon of butter for 3 to 4 minutes. Set aside on top of corn kernels. Chop raw potatoes with skin on into ½ inch chunks. Set aside on top of corn kernels as well.

Make a roux by combining flour and butter with a whisk in a medium saucepan on medium-high heat. Add salt and pepper to roux paste. Add hot vegetable broth and whisk briskly, then pour into a Dutch oven or large 8 qt. pot. Heat coconut crème in the same saucepan.

Combine corn kernels, sautéed veggies, potatoes, and hot coconut crème the roux/vegetable broth mixture, and bay leaves. After these ingredients have boiled on a low simmer for 5 minutes, add macadamia milk very slowly. Add more salt and pepper to taste. Chop the remaining cobs in half and toss them into the pot with chowder. Boil on a low simmer for 15 minutes. Remove the cobs and taste the soup's level of doneness and seasoning. Add more spice or salt and pepper to taste. Garnish in separate bowls with a basil topping. Serves 6.

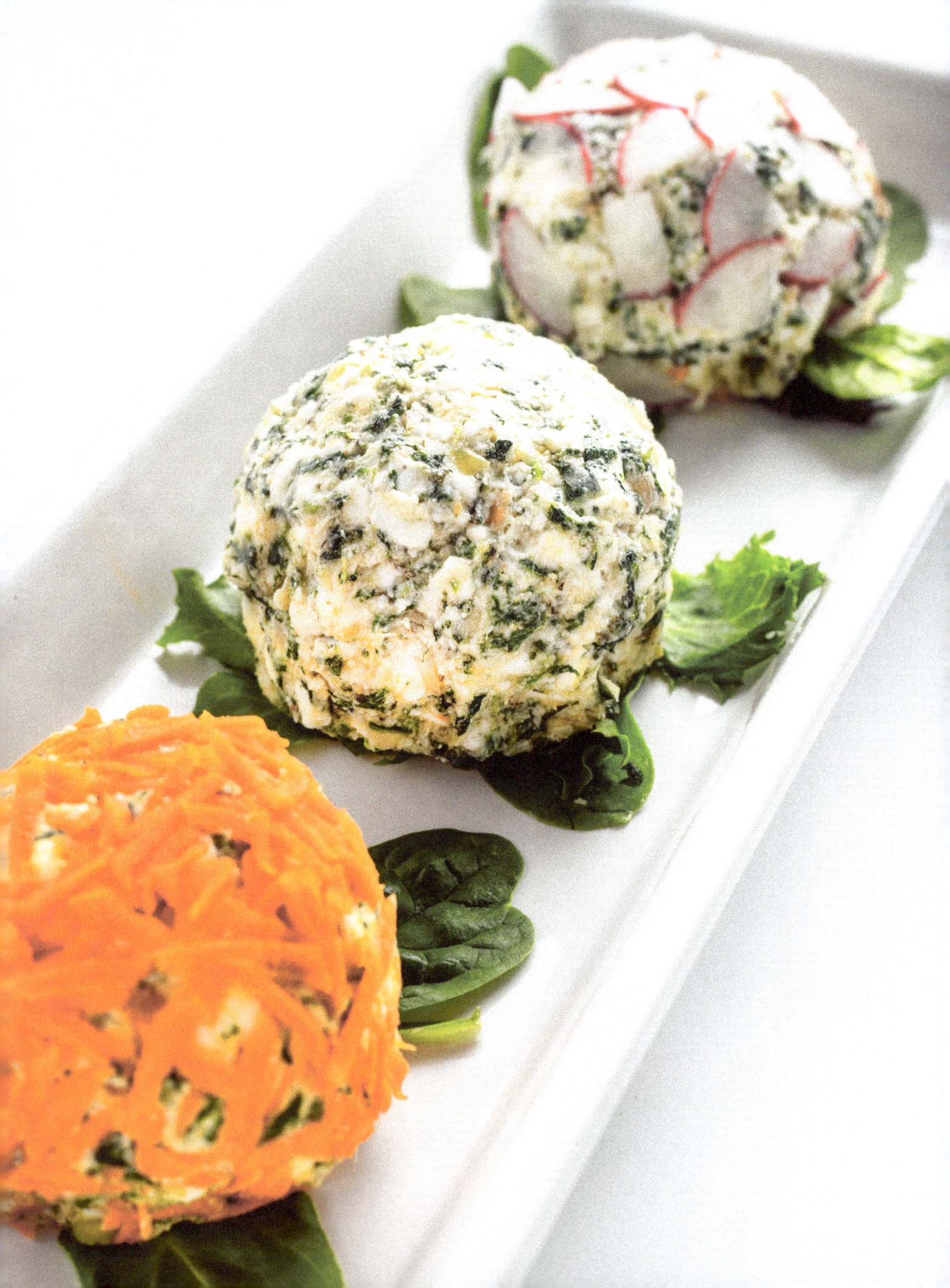

Chef Frances' Famous Feta Cheeseballs

Equipment: Large mixing bowl, cutting board, cheese knife or chef knife, cheesecloth, big mixing fork or regular fork

1½ package of Violife Feta Style cheese

2 containers of Trader Joe's Vegan Cream Cheese

8 cloves of roasted garlic, finely minced

4 cups of baby spinach

½ cup finely chopped artichoke from the jar (with or without oil)

¼ cup of vegan mayo

1 teaspoon of Louisiana Hot Sauce

1 teaspoon of garlic salt

1 teaspoon of black pepper

Directions:

Dice the feta into ¼-inch pieces with a large knife or cheese knife. Transfer to a medium-sized mixing bowl and add two containers of cream cheese. Mix with a large fork or spatula.

Cook spinach on stove top until reduced to about one cup. Drain and squeeze the water with a cheesecloth, chop, and set aside.

Add ½ of the chopped spinach and ½ of the artichoke mixture to the cheeses. Mix, then add ½ of the mayo and mix again. Keep smashing and mixing the cheeses and ingredients. Add the other half of the spinach, artichoke, and mayo, and mix again.

Add the remaining seasonings and ingredients and mix again. Refrigerate covered for at least 2 hours.

Remove the bowl from the fridge and form three balls that are approximately the size of a traditional cheese ball, about the size of a softball. You can roll the balls in almost any topping to make them look festive. I like using fried beetroot shreds, grated carrots, or ground or sliced nuts of any type. Pine nuts are super delish.

Serve with pita, bagel chips, crackers, sliced peppers, or cucumbers. You can pair the cheeseballs with anything savory, but most successfully with a Mediterranean- or Italian-themed dipper of some sort.
Serves 12 to 20 people as an appetizer. Leftovers are amazing to spread on almost anything. Incredibly versatile.

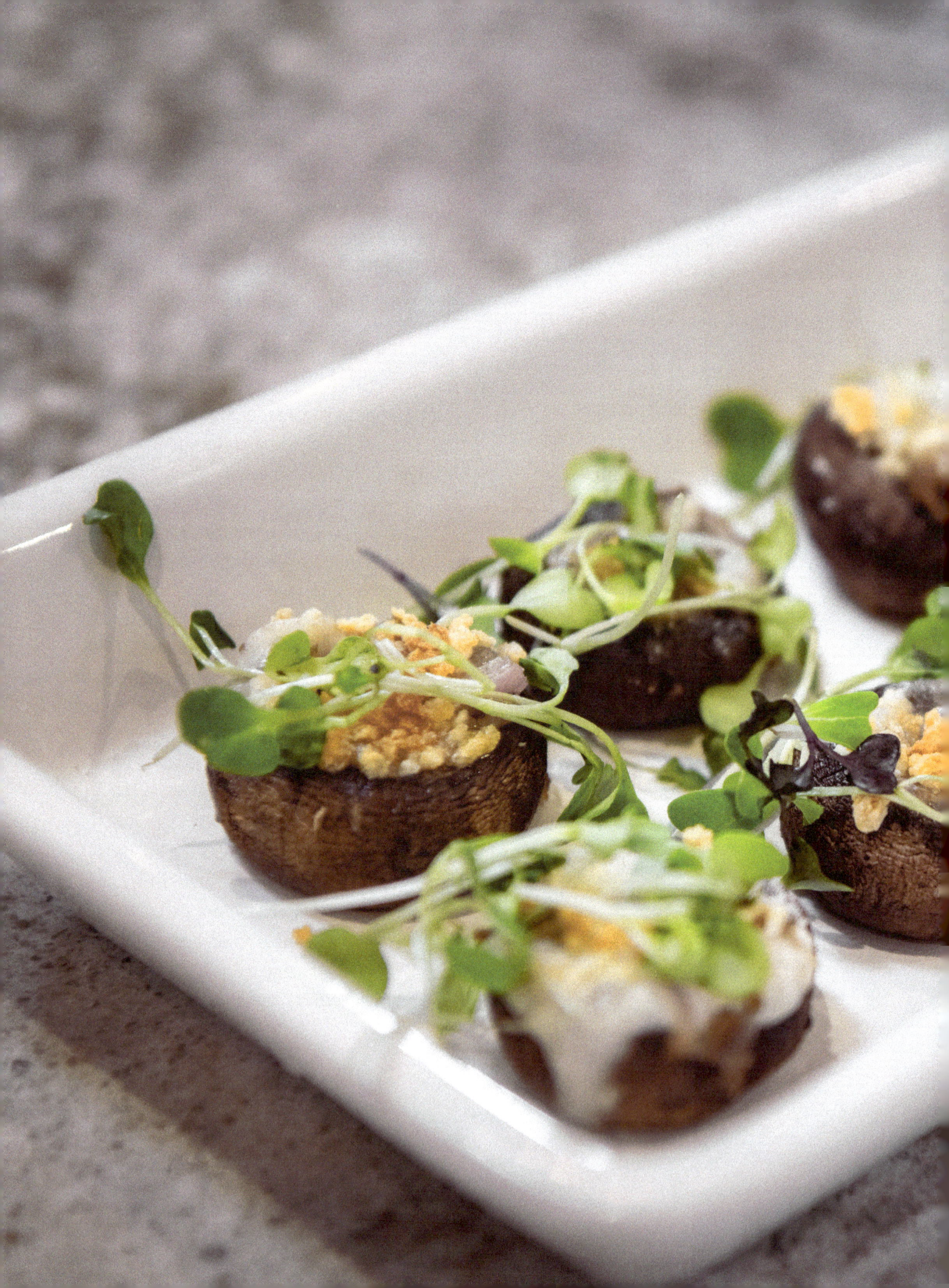

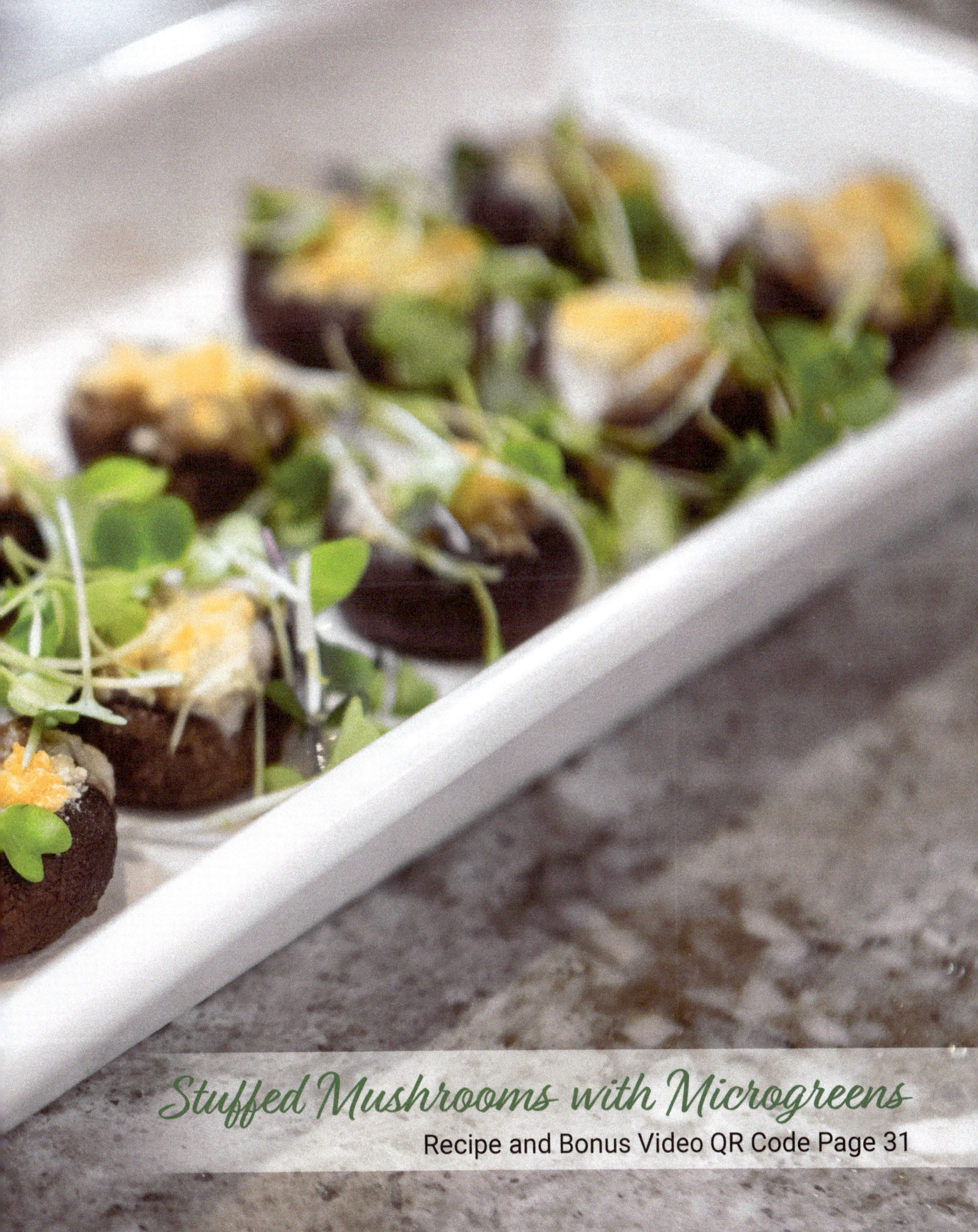

Stuffed Mushrooms with Microgreens
Recipe and Bonus Video QR Code Page 31

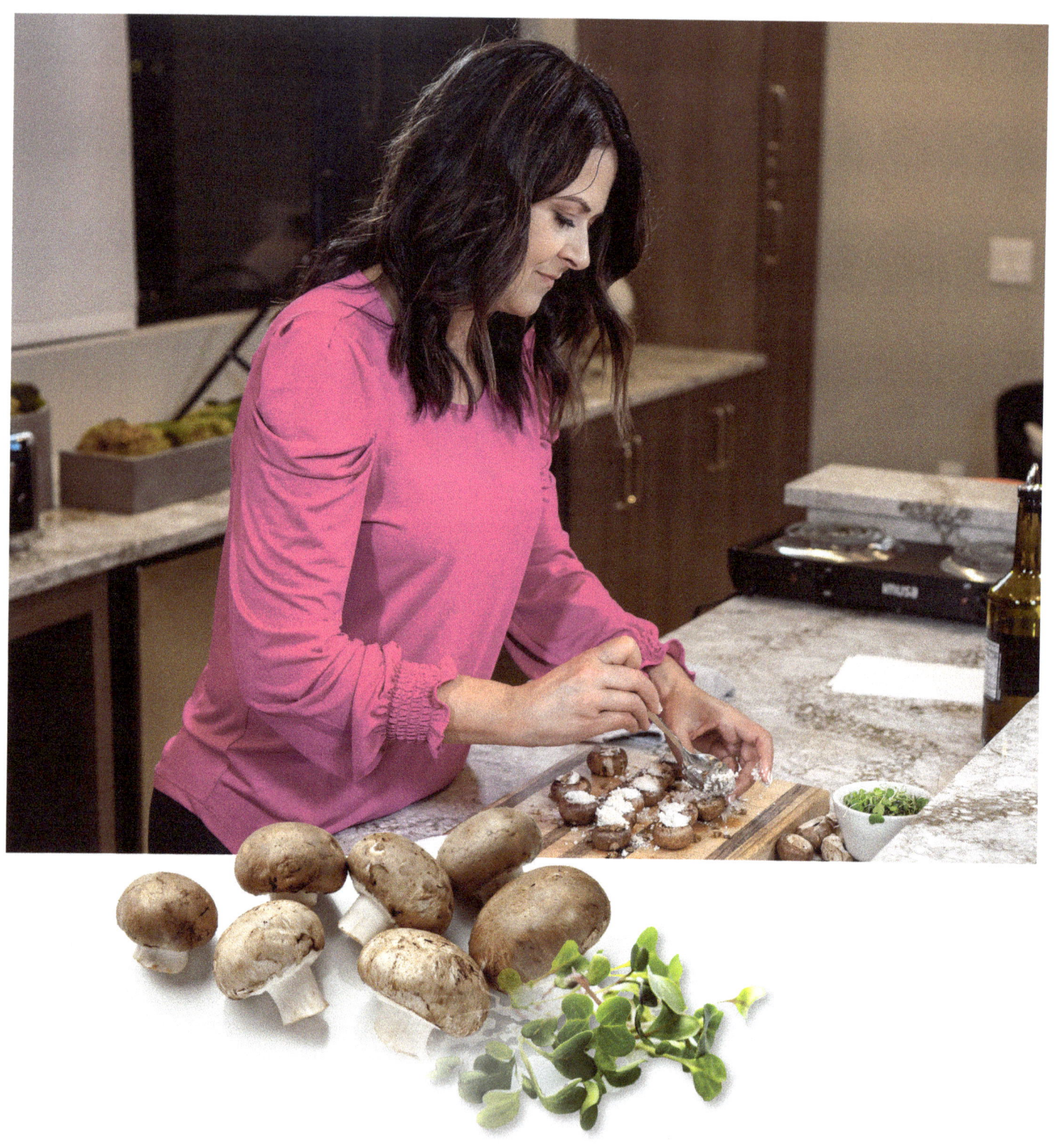

Stuffed Mushrooms with Microgreens

Equipment: Cookie sheet, medium mixing bowl, mini parchment baking cups

12 medium-sized baby portobello or cremini mushroom caps, cleaned with damp paper towels

6 tablespoons of Boursin Dairy-Free Garlic and Herb cheese alternative

4 tablespoons of gluten-free Ian's Panko breadcrumbs

½ cup of finely minced mushroom stalks

Optional: 1 drop of mushroom extract like the brand 11:11 in each mushroom cap

2 tablespoons of extra virgin olive oil

4 cloves of fresh garlic, grated

2 shallots finely minced

½ cup of microgreens

Directions:

Pre-cook the mushroom caps by making sure they are patted dry, drizzled with 1 tablespoon of olive oil, and patted dry again after roasting. Roast in an air fryer or oven for 6 minutes at 425°F.

In a small saucepan on the stove, add ½ tablespoon of olive oil, garlic, and shallots. Cook on medium-low for 4 minutes. Remove ingredients from the pan and set aside in a small bowl.

Combine mushroom stalks, Boursin cheese, 2 tablespoons of breadcrumbs, mushroom extract, and heated garlic mixture in a small mixing bowl.

Stuff pre-cooked mushrooms with the above-combined mixture. Top the mushroom caps with the remaining breadcrumbs, ½ teaspoon each.

Drizzle the remaining ½ tablespoon of olive oil sparingly over each mushroom cap. Bake at 450°F for 6 more minutes. Top with microgreens and serve in mini parchment baking cups. Serves 4 to 6.

Bonus VIDEO TUTORIAL

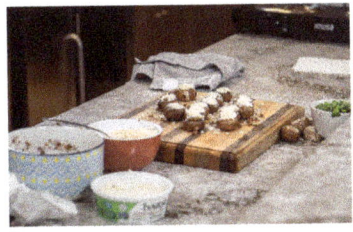

Password: Z1977Fsg1111$
Note: Save the password to your browser for easier access

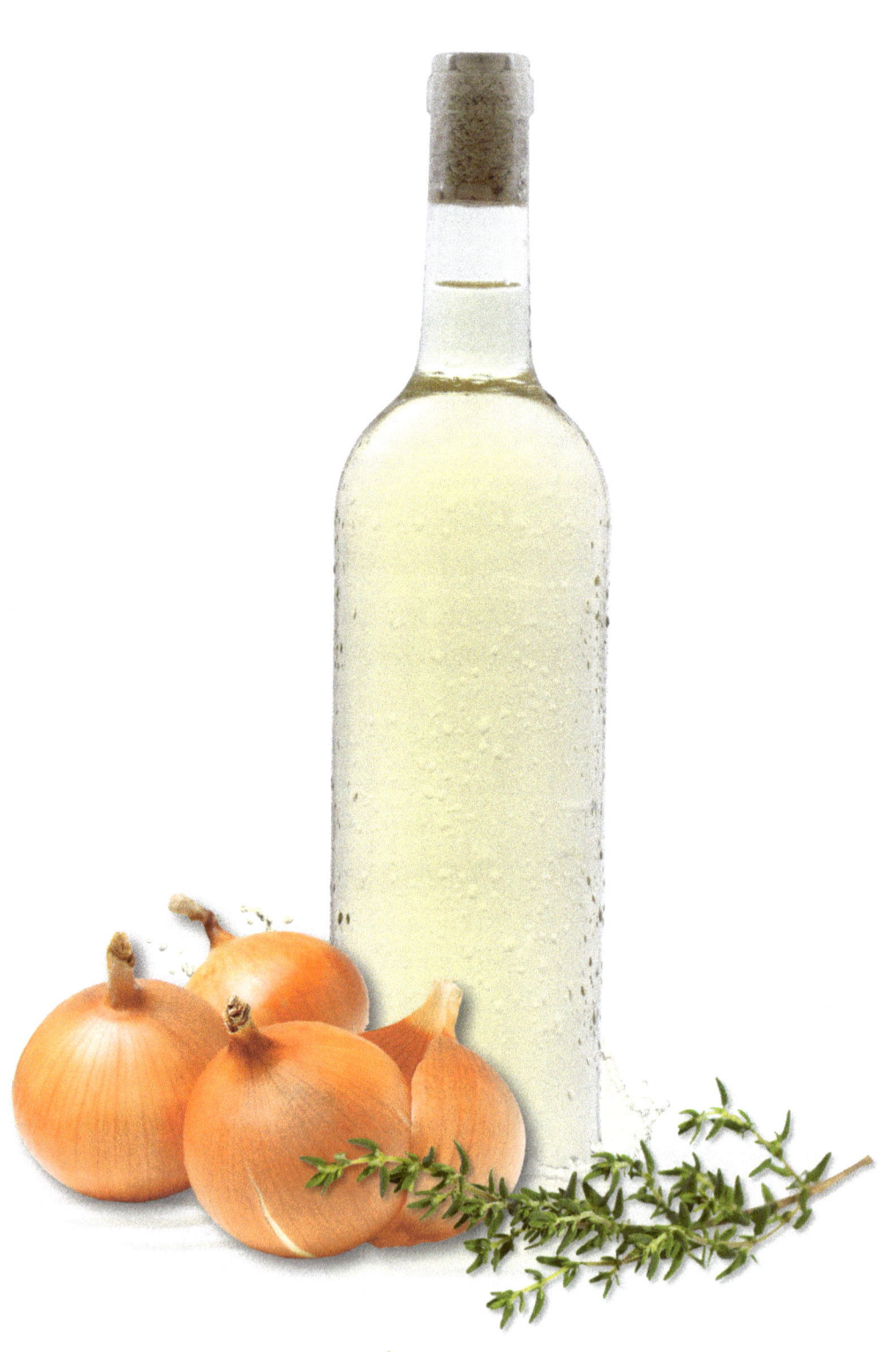

French Onion Soup

Equipment: Dutch oven or large 8 qt. pot, food processor

6 medium onions sliced with a food processor

1 tablespoon of avocado oil

4 tablespoons of Miyoko's vegan butter

2 bay leaves

2 anise seeds

1 teaspoon of mushroom powder

1 tablespoon of vegan Worcestershire sauce*

¼ teaspoon of crushed red pepper

½ teaspoon of kosher salt

½ teaspoon of black pepper

6 sprigs of fresh thyme, plus 6 for garnish

1 cup of white wine

8 cups of vegetable broth (2 4-qt. cartons)

Optional: 6 small slices of ciabatta bread (or firm bread of your choice), one slice of vegan cheese (of your choice) per bowl – I like smoked provolone cheese from Violife Foods

Directions:

Add sliced onions to butter and avocado oil. Add salt, pepper, crushed red pepper, anise seeds, and bay leaves. Cook down on medium-high heat for 20 minutes. Keep turning the onions every 3 to 4 minutes.

Add wine and turn up the heat for 5 minutes to let the alcohol evaporate. Add mushroom powder and Worcestershire sauce. Add vegetable broth and whole thyme sprigs. Turn down the heat to maintain a low simmer. Simmer for 10 minutes. Serves 6.

Optional: Scoop soup into serving bowls that are oven safe. Place a piece of ciabatta (or gluten-free ciabatta) and stack two slices of cheese in each bowl. Put all bowls on a cookie sheet and broil the bread and cheese tops for 2 to 4 minutes. Check on them every minute or so to ensure they don't burn.

Remove from oven and add one fresh thyme sprig to each bowl for garnish.
Serve immediately.

*Gluten-free vegan Worcestershire sauce is available online or at specialty health stores.

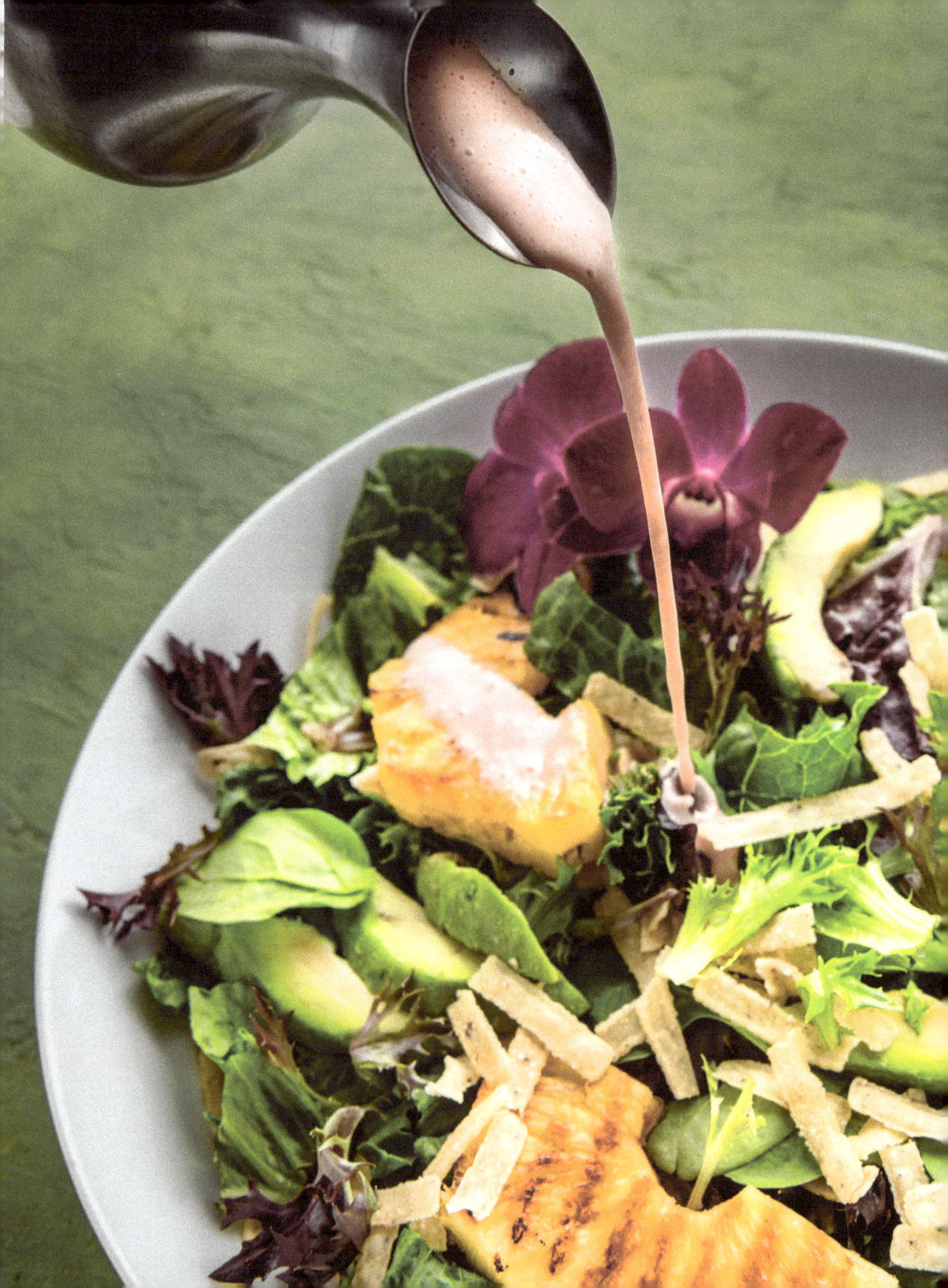

Star Salads

Not Your Typical Salads

Caesar Pasta Salad with Baby Kale, Spinach and Cashew Caesar Dressing

Sweet Potato Bowl with High-Protein Pink Dressing

Pineapple and Avocado Salad with Creamy Pomegranate Dressing

Cauliflower Power Side Salad with Agave Mustard Dressing

Cold Angel Hair Pasta Salad with Aromatic Italian Dressing

Grape Quinoa Salad with Coconut Crème, Balsamic Dressing

Israeli Couscous and Kale Salad with a Mouthwatering Vinaigrette

Broccoli Salad with Sweet and Tangy Dressing

Featured Opposite Page:

Pineapple and Avocado Salad with Creamy Pomegranate Dressing

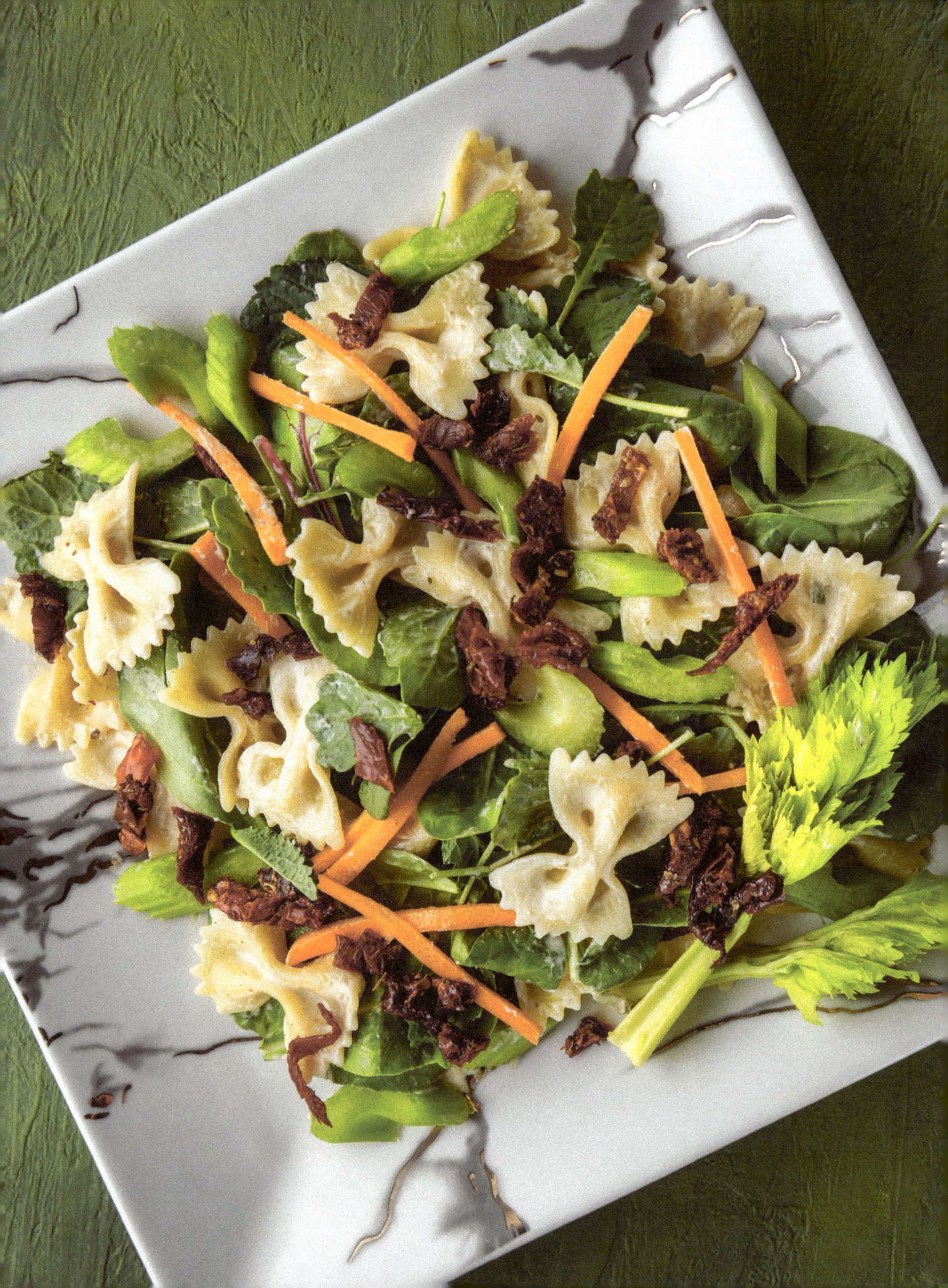

Caesar Pasta Salad with Baby Kale, Chard and Spinach with Cashew Caesar Dressing

Equipment: Large mixing bowl, chef knife or chopping device

1 lb. bowtie pasta or sweet potato pasta for gluten-free, cooked and cooled

3 stalks of celery, cut on the diagonal

1 cup of carrots, julienned (thin-cut strips)

4 cups baby kale, spinach, and chard (Trader Joe's has a mix in one bag or use fresh)

½ cup sun-dried tomatoes, finely chopped

Cashew Caesar Dressing

Equipment: Blender, large mixing bowl

1 cup of raw cashews soaked overnight in the fridge with 3 cups of water

4 roasted garlic cloves

2 tablespoons of vegan mayo

1 tablespoon of red wine vinegar

1 teaspoon of Himalayan salt

1 teaspoon of white pepper

1 tablespoon of nutritional yeast

1 teaspoon dried sweet basil

½ cup of cold water

1 tablespoon of extra virgin olive oil

2 tablespoons of freshly squeezed lemon juice

Directions:

After soaking the cashews overnight, drain the soaking liquid and set aside.

Cook pasta according to package directions, minus 2 minutes. Drain and set aside to cool.

Prepare all veggies according to the above directions. Set aside.

Take drained cashews and all other dressing ingredients and blend them in a food processor or blender; I prefer my Vitamix.

Even if the dressing seems like a lot, add it to the pasta and veggies, except the baby kale and greens. Combine. Let sit in the fridge for at least two hours before serving. Add baby kale and greens, mix lightly, and serve cold.

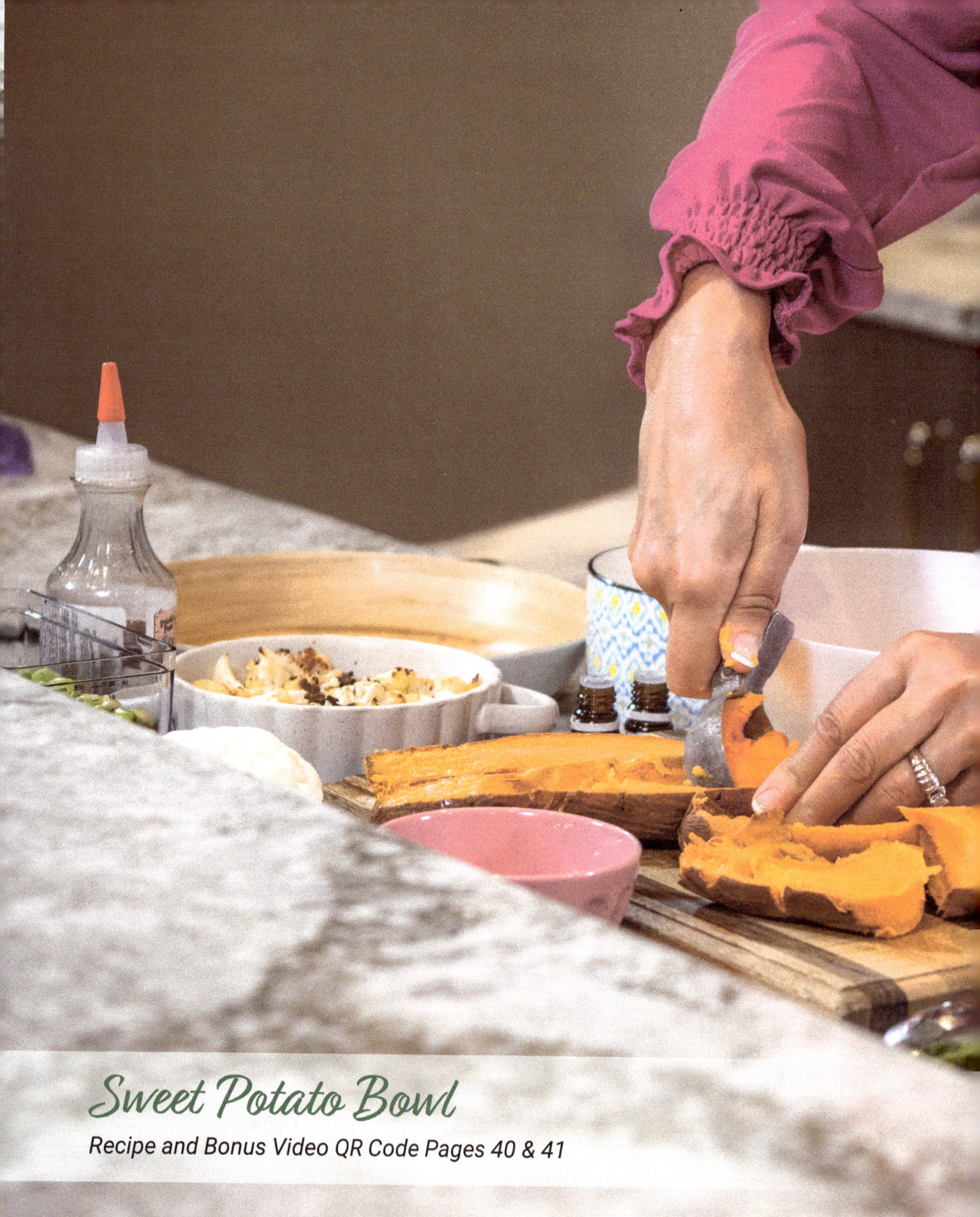

Sweet Potato Bowl

Recipe and Bonus Video QR Code Pages 40 & 41

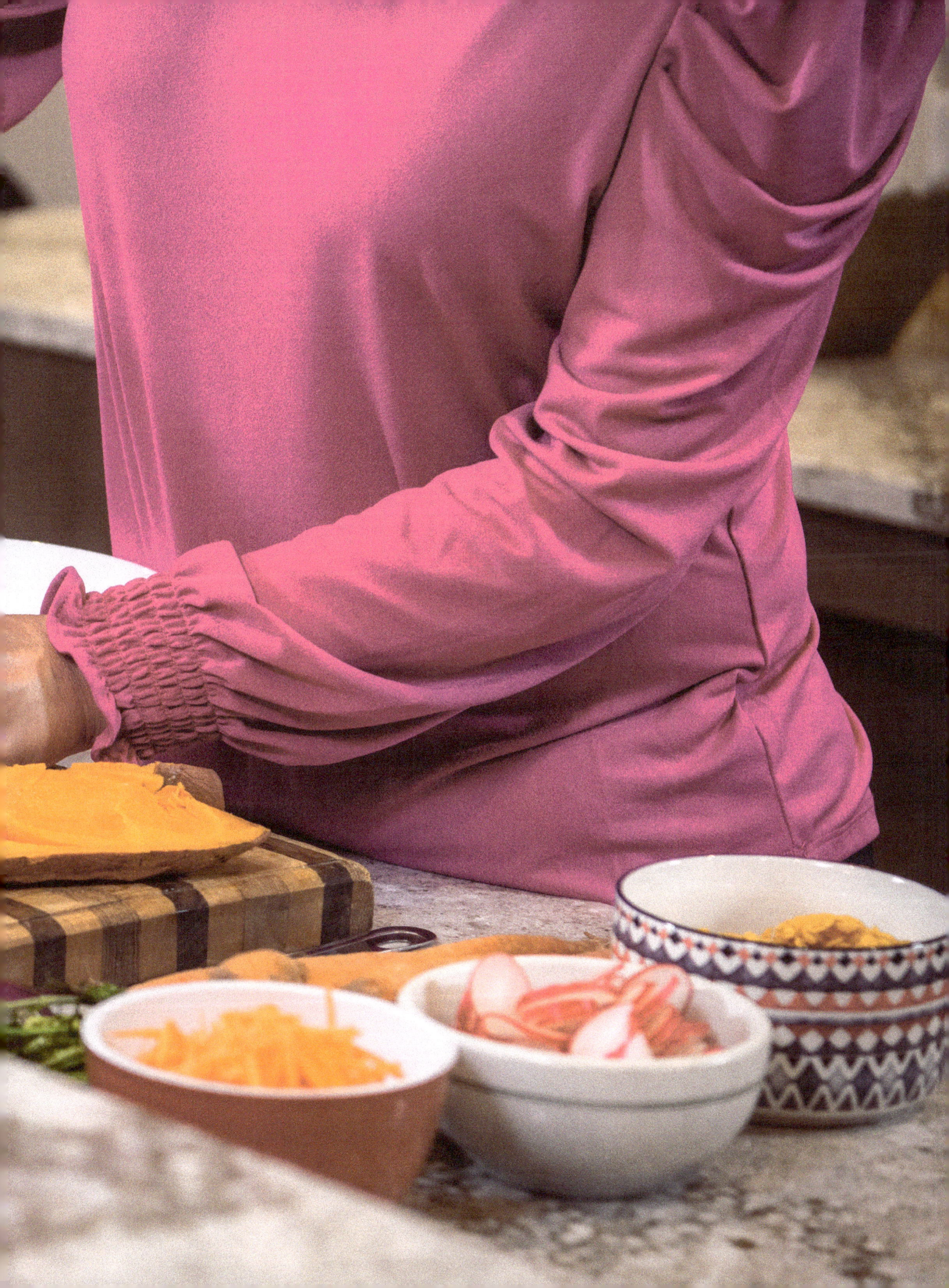

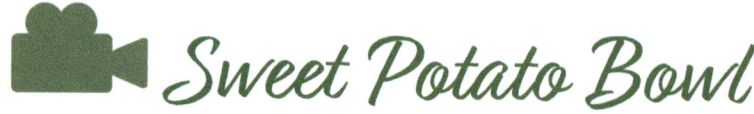

Sweet Potato Bowl
with High-Protein Pink Dressing

Equipment: Cookie sheet, medium cooking pot, chef knife or mandolin

2 large sweet potatoes, baked and mashed

1 teaspoon of Himalayan salt

½ teaspoon of white pepper

1 teaspoon of ground cinnamon

½ teaspoon of nutmeg, freshly grated

1 drop of Young Living Cardamon essential oil, or ⅛ teaspoon of cardamom (optional)

2 cups of frozen edamame, blanched

2 tablespoons of kosher salt

2 cups of carrots, julienned or shredded

2 cups of cauliflower, roasted

½ cup of pumpkin seeds

2 cups roasted zucchini, diced

1 cup of sliced, cold radishes

3 tablespoons of extra virgin olive oil

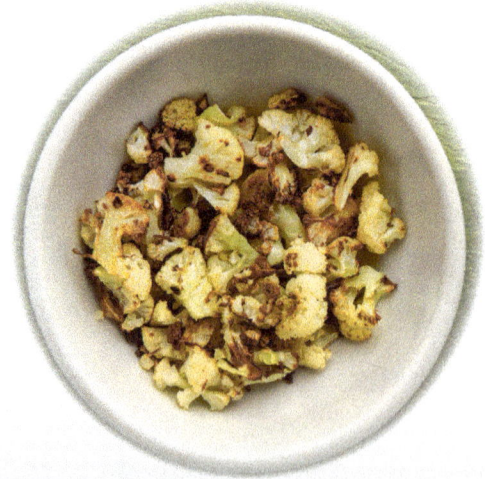

Roasted Cauliflower

Directions:

Bake sweet potatoes for 30 minutes wrapped in parchment paper-lined foil at 375°F. Remove from oven and see if they are fork tender. If not, bake for another 10 minutes. The cooking time depends on the size of the potatoes. Remove from oven and let cool. Chop into big chunks and mash with a potato masher until you get a creamy potato mash. Add the seasonings and taste for a mildly seasoned mash.

Next, roast all the veggies requiring roasting for 15 minutes at 425°F. Separate the veggies in rows on a cookie sheet so that they do not mix. Toss with 3 tablespoons of olive oil.

Blanche the edamame for 3 minutes by boiling in water with 2 tablespoons of kosher salt. Remove from water and cool in ice water.

Chop the remaining cold vegetables and set aside in separate bowls. Also, set aside the cooked vegetables in separate bowls, and the same for the pumpkin seeds.

Layering begins! In a medium bowl or plate, lay the mashed sweet potatoes and 2 tablespoons (or less) of each veggie and the seeds in a pinwheel row around and on top of the mash. Drizzle with high-protein dressing.

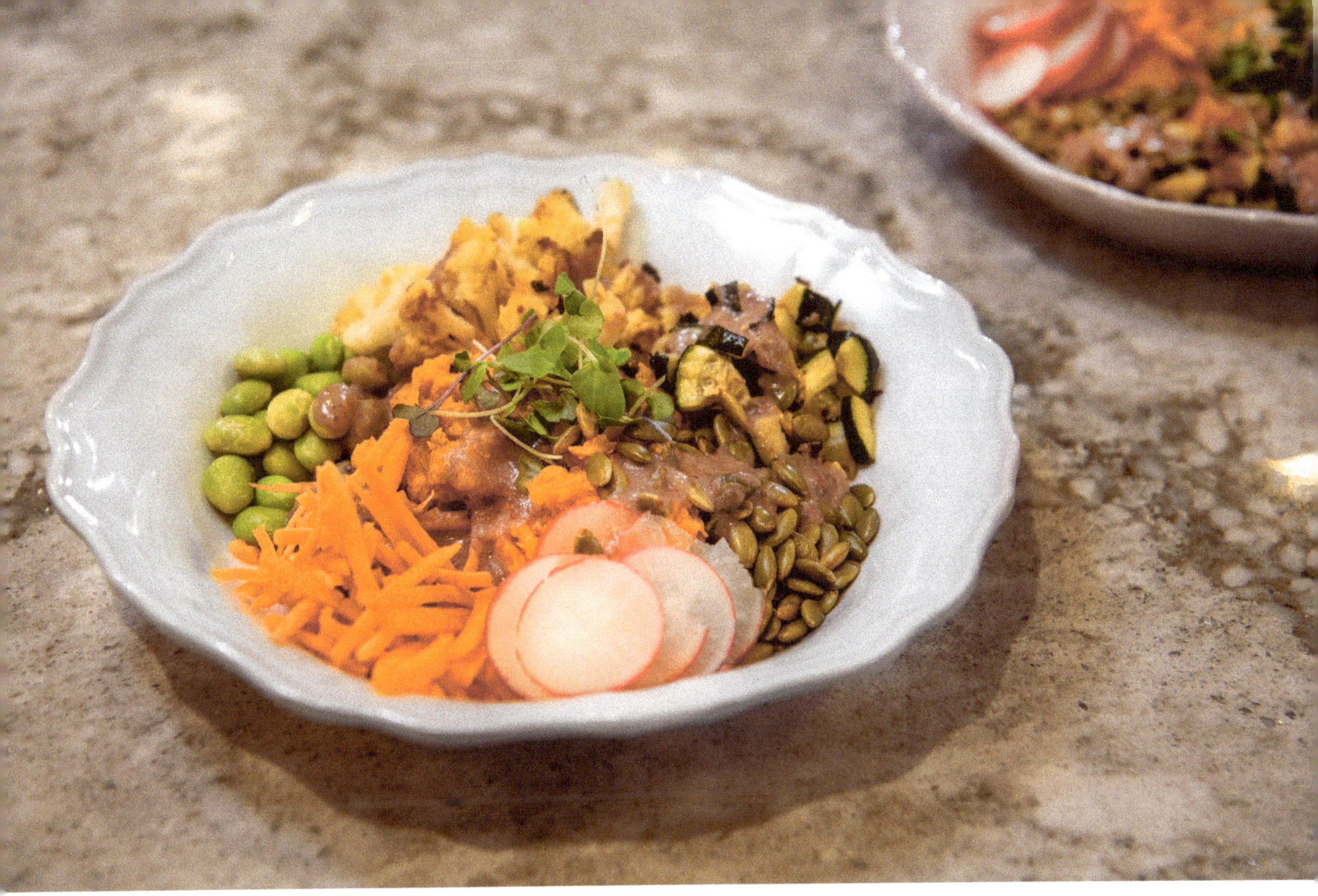

High-Protein Pink Dressing

Equipment: Blender

1 cup of cooked red lentils

2 tablespoons of dried cranberries

1 tablespoon white wine vinegar

1 teaspoon extra virgin olive oil

3 kalamata olives, pitted

Optional: 1–2 drops of Young Living Lemon
    Vitality essential oil, or any food-grade
    lemon essential oil

2 tablespoons of prickly pear syrup

1 tablespoon of monk fruit sugar

½ tablespoon of Himalayan salt

¼ cup cold water

½ teaspoon white pepper

Directions:

Blend all ingredients in a blender.
Chill for at least 2 hours. Blend again
after chilling. Serve as a salad dressing
or versatile sauce.

Bonus VIDEO TUTORIAL

 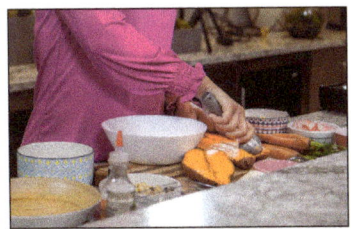

Password: Z1977Fsg1111$

Note: Save the password to your browser
for easier access

Pineapple and Avocado Salad
with Creamy Pomegranate Dressing

Equipment: Indoor or outdoor grill, small saucepan, chef knife

4 cups of chopped organic romaine lettuce

4 cups of spring greens

8 pineapple rings, grilled (when grilling, baste with a combination of dark rum and organic brown sugar, ¼ cup of each)

2 large avocados, sliced

1 tablespoon of fresh lime juice

1 cup of organic white or yellow corn tortilla strips

1 teaspoon of Tajin

1 tablespoon of kosher salt

Optional: 1 medium red onion sliced into thin rings, edible orchid garnish

Directions:

Fire up the grill! Lay the pineapple rings on the grill to cook as well. Baste them with the rum mixture. Flip after 3 minutes and baste the other side. Turn one last time and remove after 2 minutes, grilling for a total of 8 minutes. Set aside.

Roughly chop lettuce and set aside. Combine spring greens with chopped lettuce and put a bottom layer of the greens and lettuce in serving bowls or large deep plates.

Cut whole tortillas into thin strips, lightly salt, and fry in avocado oil or air fry with cooking spray. Lightly cover the strips with coconut oil cooking spray and fry for 6 minutes. Remove, lightly salt, and set aside.

Cut the avocados in half and slice each half inside the rind. Drizzle lime juice on and salt each avocado section. Set aside and keep in the rind until dressing is created.

Creamy Pomegranate Dressing

Equipment: Blender or blender cup

¾ cup fresh pomegranate juice

1½ tablespoons of champagne vinegar

1 tablespoon fresh lime juice

¼ cup of avocado oil

1 tablespoon cilantro, finely minced

1 teaspoon organic onion powder

1 teaspoon kosher salt

1 teaspoon black pepper

1 tablespoon of organic unbleached cane sugar

2 tablespoons of vegan mayo

¼ cup of blue agave syrup

Directions:

Combine all ingredients in a blender or with a mini-mixing attachment. Feel free to double or triple the above ingredients. Chill for 2 hours before serving for an even more flavorful-tasting dressing.

Layer the lettuce and spring greens at the bottom of your salad plate as stated above. Next, layer the avocado and 2 pineapple rings on each bowl or plate. If you add the red onion rings, put them in a pattern around the plate. Lastly, sprinkle the Tajin on the tortilla strips, then layer the strips over the salad and add the dressing.

Serves 4.

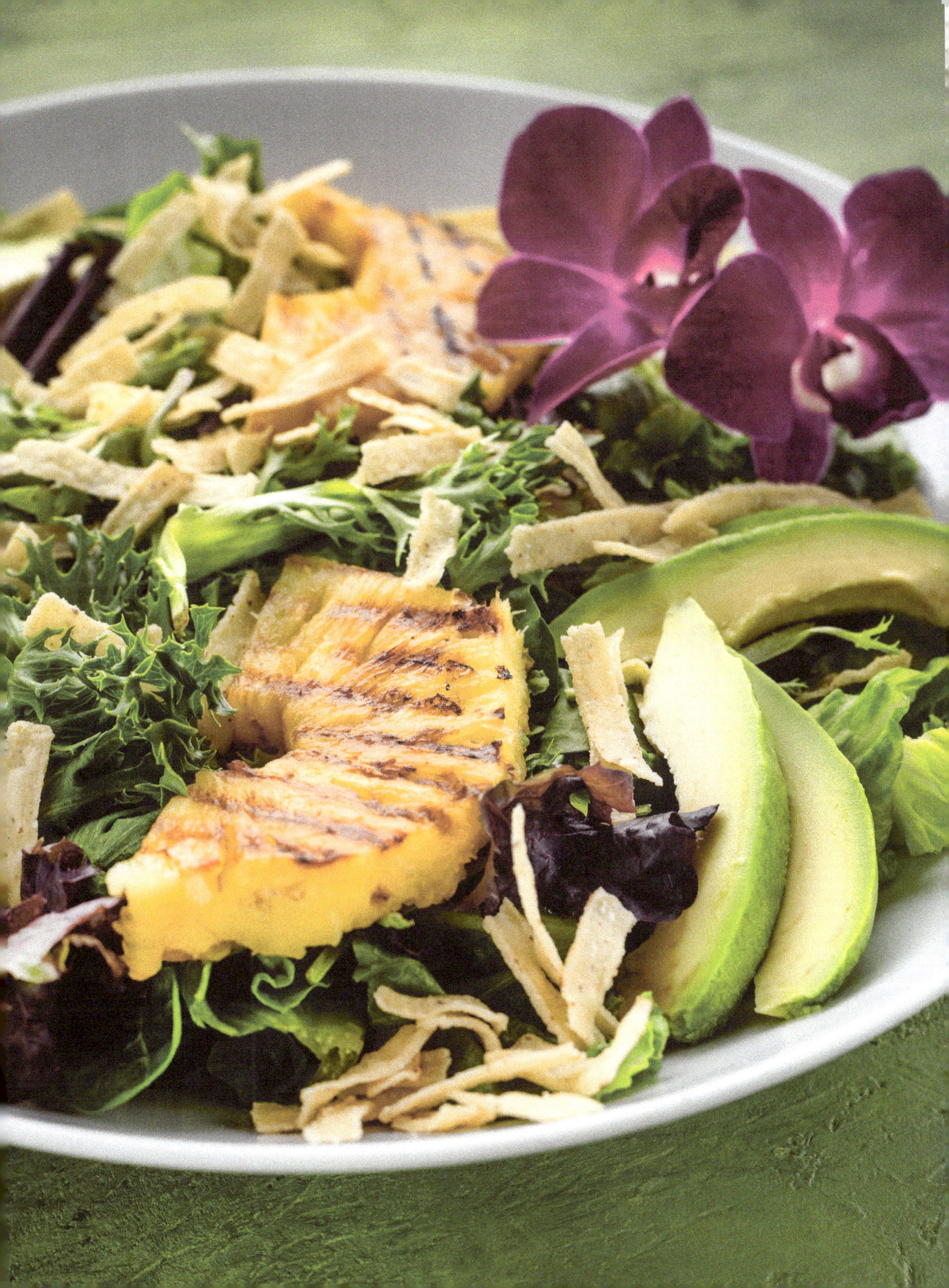

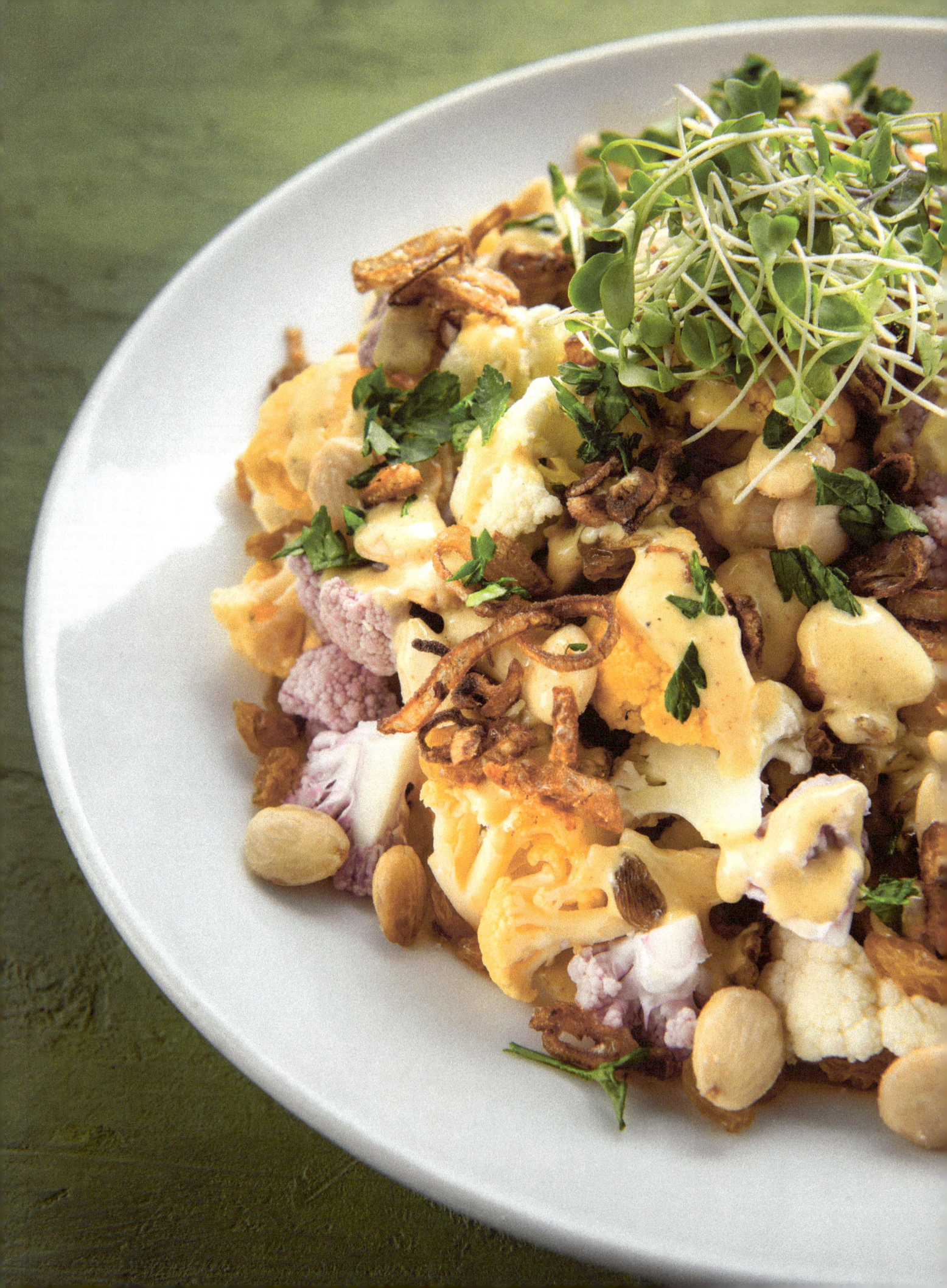

Cauliflower Power Side Salad
with Agave Mustard Dressing

Equipment: Large mixing bowl, large serving bowl (can be the same bowl), chef knife or chopper

1 head each of orange, purple, and white organic cauliflower

1 cup of Marcona almonds

1 cup of golden raisins

1 cup of celery, finely diced

1 cup of shallots, sliced into rings

1–1½ cups of avocado oil (for frying)

½ cup of flat-leaf parsley, freshly minced

Agave Mustard Dressing

Equipment: Blender cup or blender

¼ cup yellow mustard

¼ cup Dijon mustard

¼ cup cold water

½ cup agave syrup

2 tablespoons of monk fruit sugar

½ cup of vegan mayo

2 tablespoons of apple cider vinegar

½ tablespoon of garlic salt

½ teaspoon of onion powder

¼ teaspoon of cayenne pepper

Directions:

Wash and chop the cauliflower into small florets.

Add ¼ cup of raw shallots to a small saucepan of avocado oil on medium-high heat and fry for 4 minutes per batch. Drain on paper towels and set aside.

In a large serving bowl, combine cauliflower florets, almonds, celery, and raisins, and toss evenly. Cover and refrigerate while making the dressing.

Make the dressing by combining the ingredients in a blender at low speed and refrigerate for at least 1 hour. Pour dressing over the salad and evenly combine. Sprinkle parsley and shallots over the top.

Serves 6 to 8.

Cold Angel Hair Pasta with Roma Tomatoes
and Aromatic Italian Dressing

Equipment: Large mixing bowl, large cooking pot, cutting board, chef knife

1 lb. of angel hair pasta or Jovial brand capellini pasta, gluten-free

8 Roma tomatoes, chopped into ½-inch chunks

1 cup of Ian's Gluten-Free Breadcrumbs, toasted

½ cup of fresh basil chiffonade

Optional: ½ cup sliced black olives and green olives or Kalamata olives

Aromatic Italian Dressing

Equipment: Blender cup or blender

½ cup of extra virgin cold-pressed olive oil

¼ cup of high-quality red wine vinegar

4 cloves of garlic, roasted

1 tablespoon of fresh lemon juice

1 teaspoon of dried oregano

1 teaspoon of fresh minced rosemary

½ teaspoon of onion powder

1 tablespoon of monk fruit sugar

1 teaspoon of kosher salt

½ teaspoon of cayenne pepper

Optional: 1 drop of Vitality Young Living Celery Seed essential oil, or food-grade celery seed essential oil of your choice

Directions:

Cook the angel hair pasta for 2 minutes less than the package directions, drain and transfer to a large serving bowl or Tupperware container and let cool for 10 minutes, then refrigerate for another 20 minutes.

Chop tomatoes and add to the pasta. Toast breadcrumbs by sautéing in a small dry saucepan on medium-high for 3 to 4 minutes. Toss the breadcrumbs while toasting to prevent burning. Add breadcrumbs to pasta and toss.

Combine all the dressing ingredients by blending them in a small blender cup. Immediately add the dressing to the cold pasta. Set aside in the fridge for at least one hour before serving.

Add sliced olives (optional) and basil chiffonade to the pasta before serving. Serves 4 to 6 as a side dish.

Basil Chiffonade Directions:

Stack 7 to 8 basil leaves and roll tightly. Gently slice each roll from end to end. The result should be spiral-shaped thin slices of basil. For this recipe, repeat this process until you get at least ½ cup of basil chiffonade.

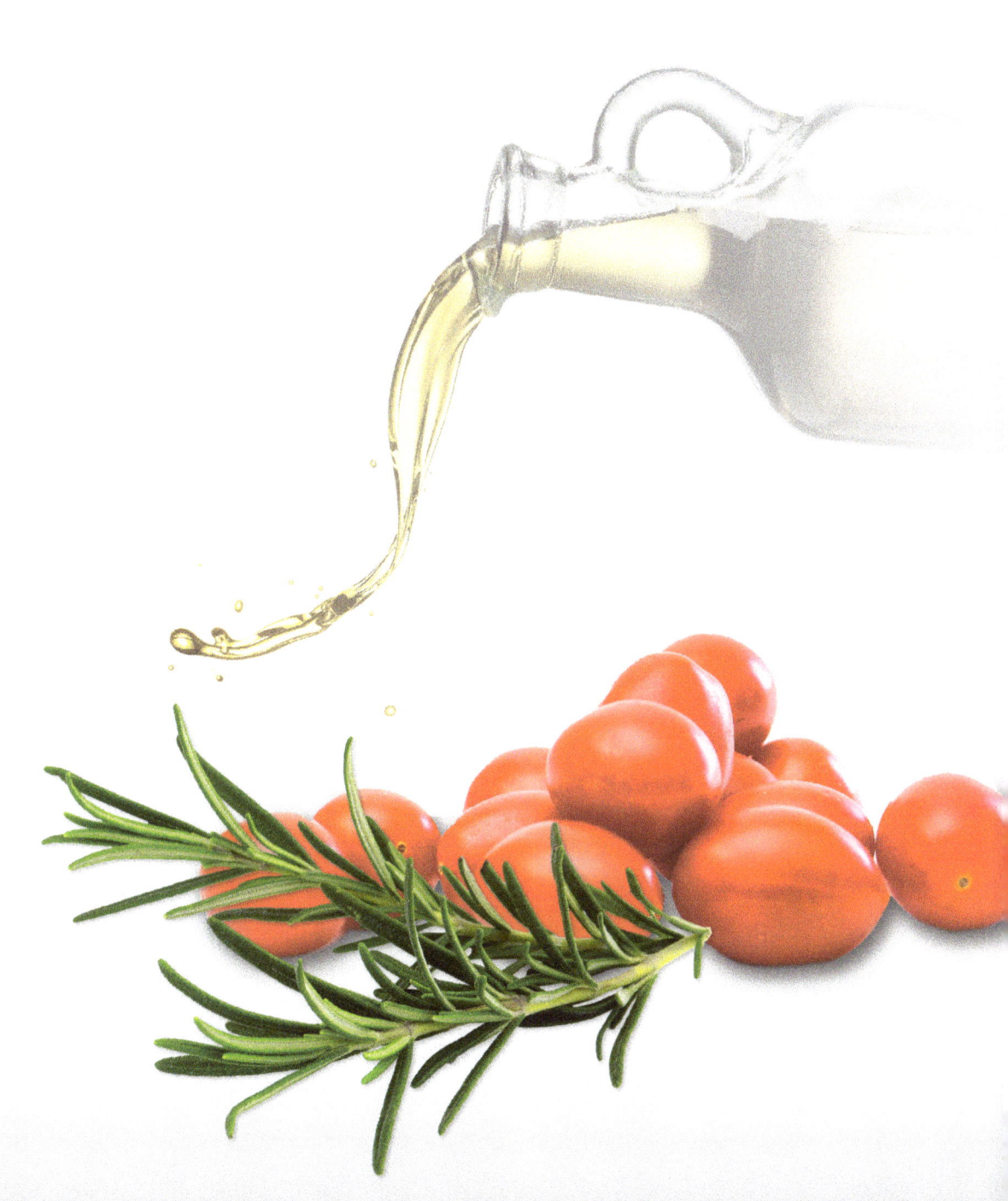

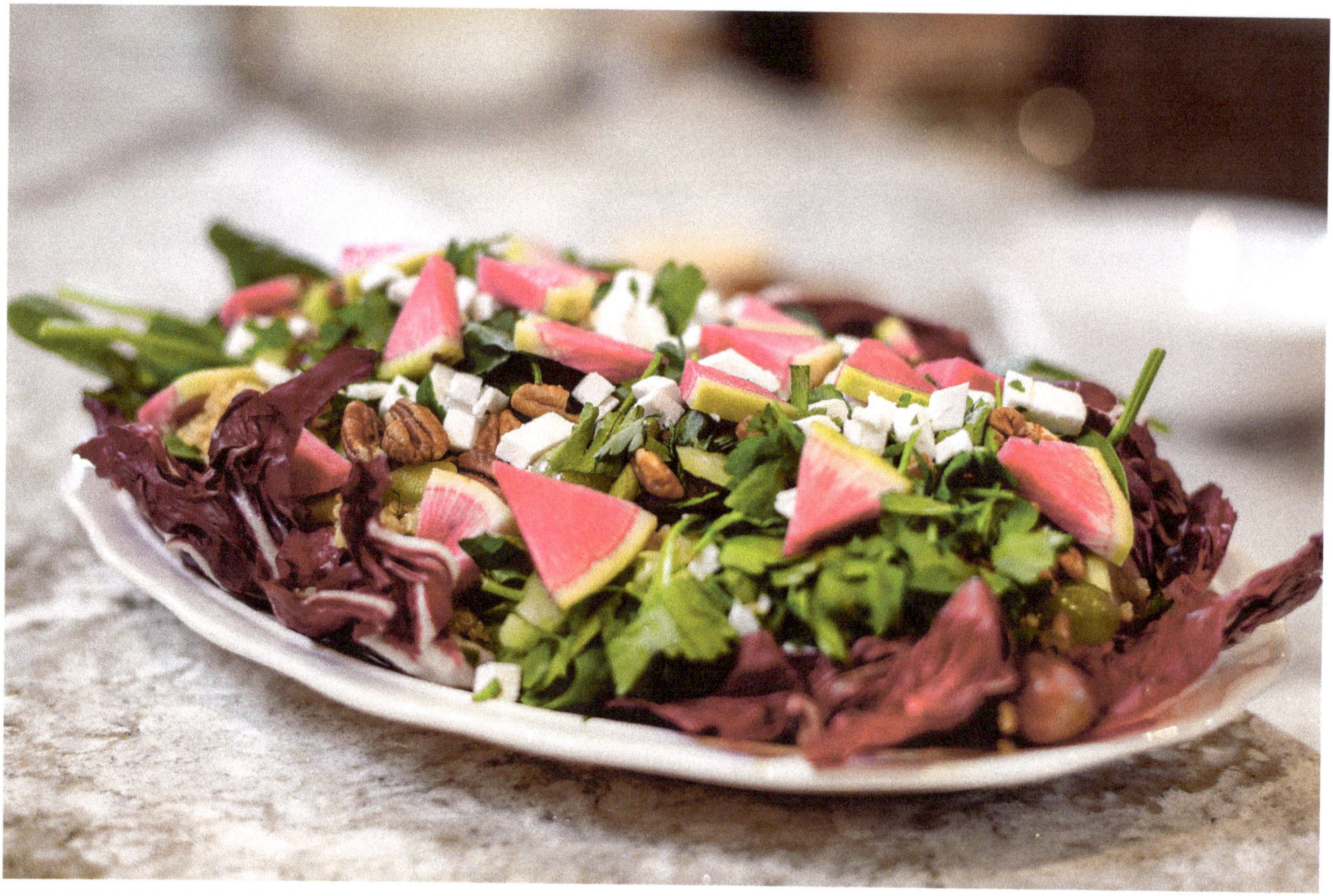

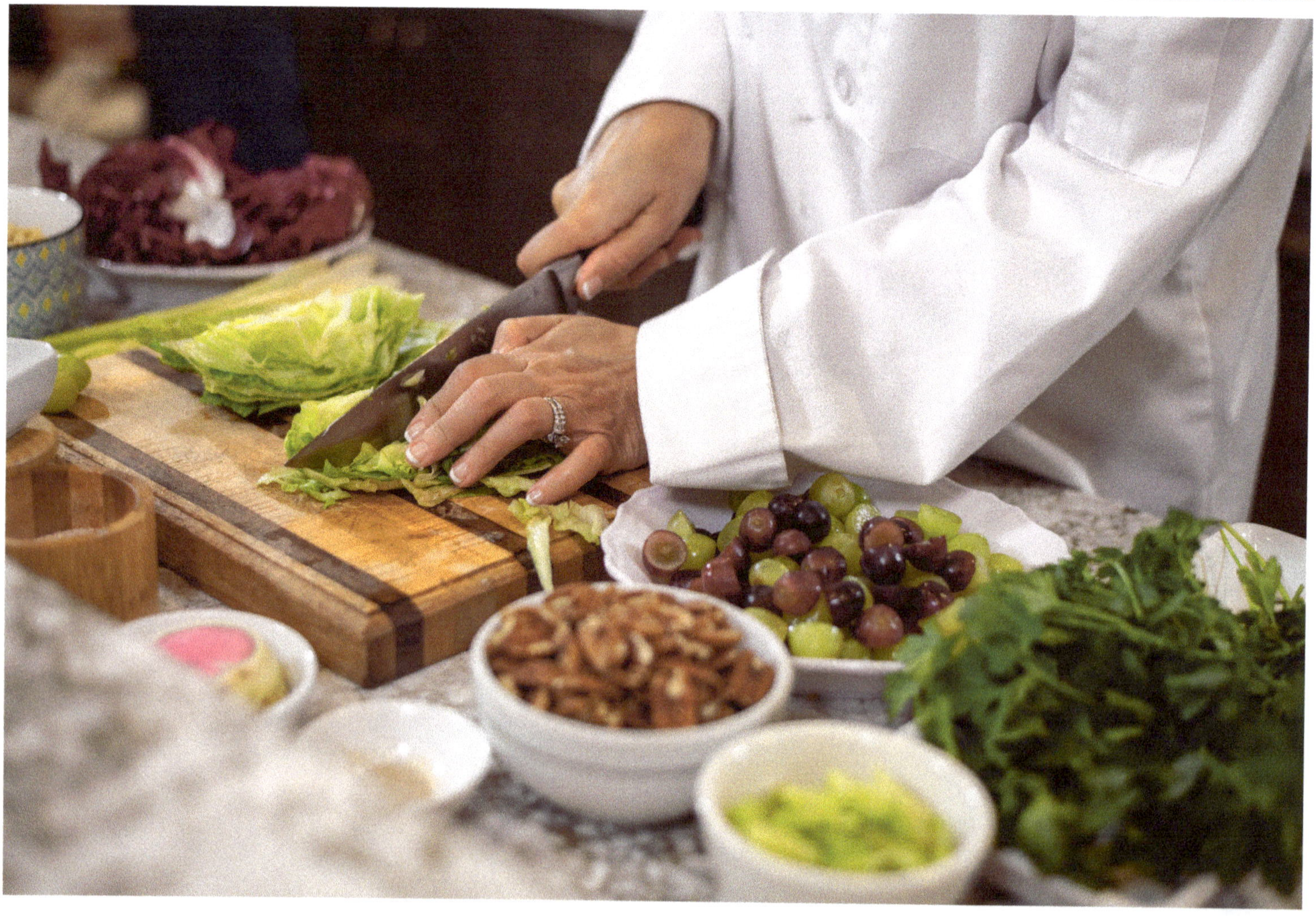

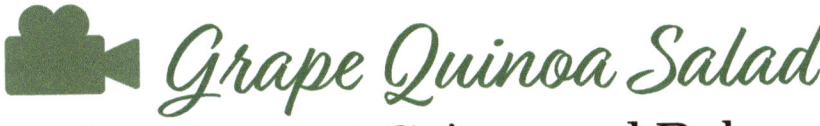

Grape Quinoa Salad
with a Coconut Crème and Balsamic Dressing

Equipment: Large mixing bowl, large serving platter or bowl, blender, medium sauté pan

4 cups of baby spinach

2 cups of radicchio

2 cups of iceberg lettuce

3 cups of white quinoa
   (cooked in vegetable broth)

3 cups of white grapes and red grapes, washed thoroughly and sliced in half

1½ cups toasted pecans, chopped

1½ cups celery, sliced diagonally

1 cup of Violife Feta, chopped finely and crumbled

Optional: 1½ cups of watermelon radish, finely sliced and halved

Coconut Crème Balsamic Dressing

2 cups of coconut crème, water drained

4 tablespoons of balsamic glaze or 4 tablespoons of balsamic vinegar cooked down for 20 minutes by simmering on low heat until reduced to a glaze (add 1 tablespoon of organic sugar)

1 teaspoon of Himalayan salt

1 teaspoon of onion powder

1 tablespoon of freshly minced flat-leaf parsley

Directions:
Combine all the ingredients except the parsley by whisking them in a medium-sized mixing bowl. Sprinkle in the parsley and use this dressing immediately. It does not keep well in the fridge because of the coconut fat, so make it fresh.

Directions:
Cook the quinoa in 4 cups of vegetable broth for 5 minutes on high, covered. Simmer quinoa for another 12 minutes on low. Drain if needed and season according to your desired level of flavor or salt and pepper lightly.

Roughly chop the spinach, radicchio, and lettuce. Lay the lettuces at the bottom of a large serving platter that has some depth, similar to a bowl. Layer the cooled quinoa on top of the lettuces. Take the halved grapes, celery, radishes, and pecans and spread them evenly on the quinoa layer. Right before serving, drizzle the dressing over the top of the salad. Toss the salad to cover the lettuce thoroughly but leave whole pieces of radicchio fanned and framed under the other lettuces. The framed radicchio can be placed around the platter or bowl before or after making the salad. Serves 6.

Bonus VIDEO TUTORIAL

 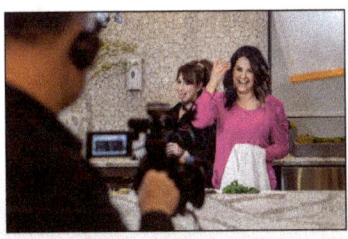

Password: Z1977Fsg1111$
Note: Save the password to your browser for easier access

Israeli Couscous and Kale Salad
with Mouthwatering Vinaigrette

Equipment: Large mixing bowl, medium pot, cutting board, chef knife or chopper

1 lb. Israeli couscous, precooked and cooled

1½ cups of fresh kale, shredded (any type)

1 cup carrots, julienned
   (available this way in most grocery stores)

½ cup watermelon radish, diced

1 cup of cooked red beets,
   diced into small cubes

½ cup shallots, finely sliced and fried

½ cup pistachios, chopped

Mouthwatering Vinaigrette Recipe

Equipment: Blender or blender cup, sauté pan or foil

2 tablespoons of Dijon mustard

2 tablespoons of organic maple syrup

½ cup champagne vinegar

¼ cup extra virgin olive oil

4 garlic cloves, roasted in the oven
   or a sauté pan on the stove

1 teaspoon of nutritional yeast

½ teaspoon of marjoram

½ teaspoon dried sweet basil

Salt and pepper to taste

Directions:

Boil couscous for 7 minutes or less, drain, and set aside to cool. Fry sliced shallots in oil for 3 to 5 minutes or until they turn slightly brown. You can also air fry them with a smaller amount of oil for the same amount of time.

Prepare vinaigrette by combining ingredients in a blender cup and set aside. Pour ¼ of the vinaigrette onto the kale. Massage kale with your hands for about a minute. Add all other ingredients including couscous, then pour the remainder of the vinaigrette on the entire salad and serve.
Feel free to add other vegetables!

Great as a side dish. Serves 4 to 6.

Broccoli Salad
with Sweet and Tangy Dressing

Equipment: Large mixing bowl/serving bowl, chef knife or food processor

1 head of fresh broccoli, roughly chopped, or organic broccoli slaw from a package

½ of one medium-sized red onion, finely chopped

½ cup of celery, finely chopped

¼ cup fresh parsley, finely minced

1 cup roasted and salted sunflower seeds or roasted cashew pieces

1 cup of dried cranberries

Sweet and Tangy Dressing

Equipment: Blender or blender cup

2 tablespoons of fresh lemon juice

¼ cup dark amber agave syrup

1 tablespoon of prickly pear syrup

¼ cup of apple cider vinegar

½ cup of extra virgin olive oil

Salt and pepper to taste, starting with ½ teaspoon each

Directions:

Roughly chop the broccoli and add to a food processor. You will end up with finely chopped broccoli and broccoli stalk; this is the consistency you are looking for.

In a large mixing bowl, add processed broccoli or broccoli slaw and the rest of the ingredients, excluding the dressing ingredients and the sunflower seeds. Toss the ingredients to evenly combine.

Add the dressing ingredients to a small blender cup and blend at high speed for 2 minutes. Pour the dressing over the salad and mix thoroughly.

Put the broccoli salad in the refrigerator for at least two hours. When you're ready to serve, add the sunflower seeds and toss one more time.

Serves 6 to 8.

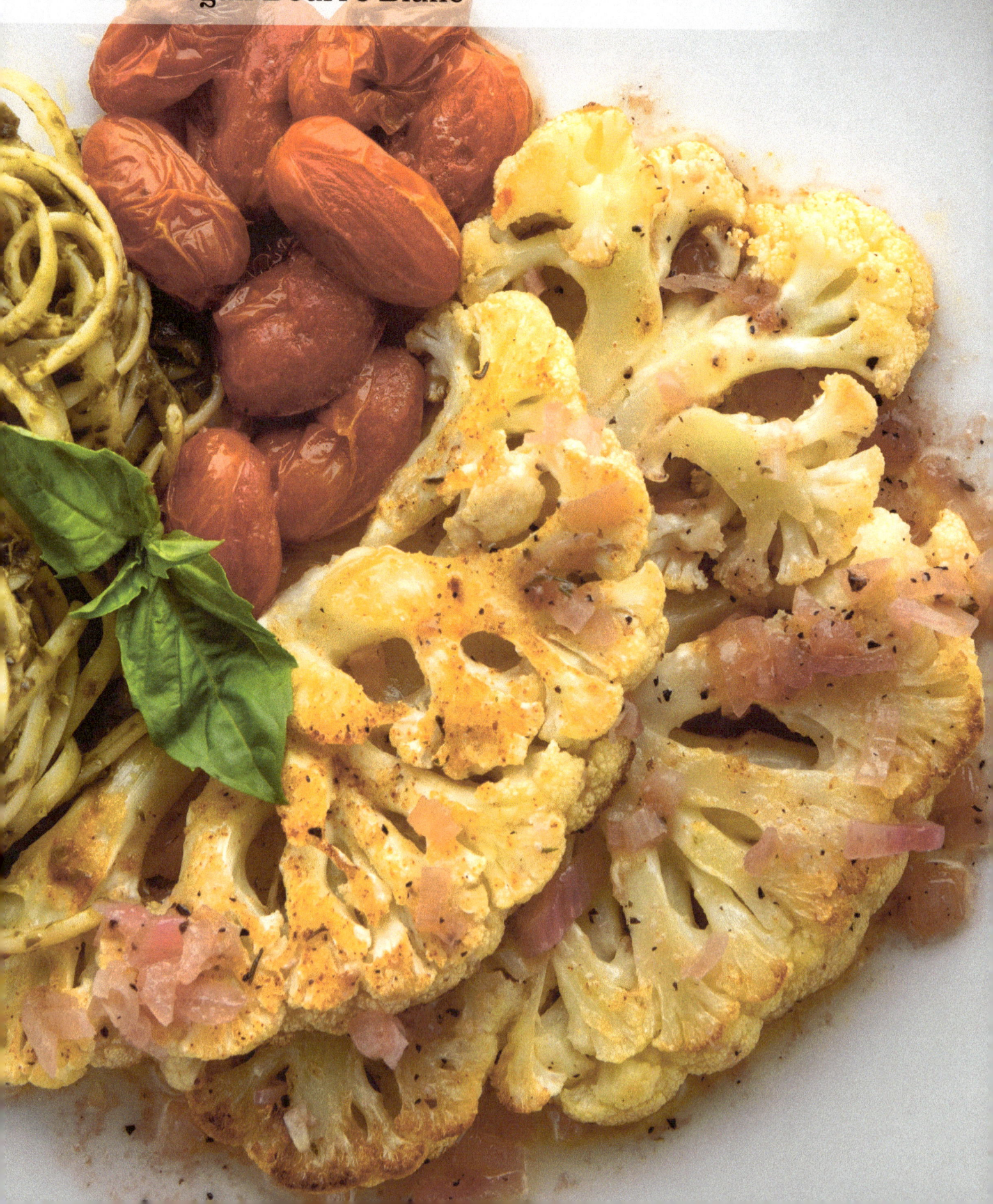

Roasted Cauliflower Steaks *Recipe Page 54*
with Vegan Beurre Blanc

Main Meals

Roasted Cauliflower Steaks with Vegan Beurre Blanc

Veggie and Daring Chicken Skewers

Breakfast Hash

Mushroom Risotto with Roasted Red Peppers and Sweet Peas

Vegan Crab Cakes

Tomato and Spinach JUST Egg Omelet

Vegan Shepherd's Pie

Carne Asada Potato Enchiladas

Stuffed Poblano Peppers with Crispy Corn Griddle Cakes and Calabacitas

Featured Opposite Page:
Roasted Cauliflower Steaks with Vegan Beurre Blanc

Roasted Cauliflower Steaks
with Vegan Beurre Blanc

Equipment: 2 large deep cookie sheets, chef knife

2 heads of cauliflower (for added color, you could use orange or purple)

½ tablespoon of sweet paprika

4 garlic cloves

1 teaspoon of smoked paprika

1 teaspoon of garlic salt

1 teaspoon of black pepper

2 tablespoons of extra virgin olive oil

Vegan Beurre Blanc

Equipment: 1 medium-sized non-stick sauté pan, whisk

6 tablespoons of Miyoko's vegan butter

2 minced shallots

½ cup dry white organic vegan wine

1 teaspoon of garlic powder or 2 fresh garlic cloves, minced

¼ cup miso broth

Directions:

Cut the cauliflower into thick slices making sure not to let the florets break off. Your goal is to have even "steak slices". Slice as many even pieces as you can and reserve the remaining florets for another recipe. Thinly slice garlic cloves and evenly lay them under each cauliflower steak on the cookie sheets.

Sprinkle seasonings evenly on cauliflower steaks and drizzle oil over the top before putting them in the oven at 375°F for 15 minutes. Turn up the heat to 425°F and cook for an additional 10 minutes. You should see a light brown to dark brown caramelization on the top of the steaks before removing them from the oven.

Ten minutes before the cauliflower steaks are done, start making the beurre blanc. Start with sautéing the butter on medium-high heat, using a whisk to move around the butter while it's melting. Add the minced shallots and sauté for 2 minutes on medium-low—turn down the heat slightly. Turn up the heat again to medium-high and add the wine. Simmer for 2 more minutes. Add the remaining ingredients. Simmer gently for an additional 6 minutes. The sauce should thicken. Add salt or pepper or both to taste.

Plate cauliflower steaks with two sides of your choice. Ladle one tablespoon of beurre blanc on top of each cauliflower steak. A starch and another colorful vegetable are good choices for two sides. Feel free to use a green garnish to brighten up the plate. I like to add pesto pasta on the side with sauteed cherry tomatoes. You can use any type of side, but the cauliflower steak is the star of this meal. Serves 4 to 6.

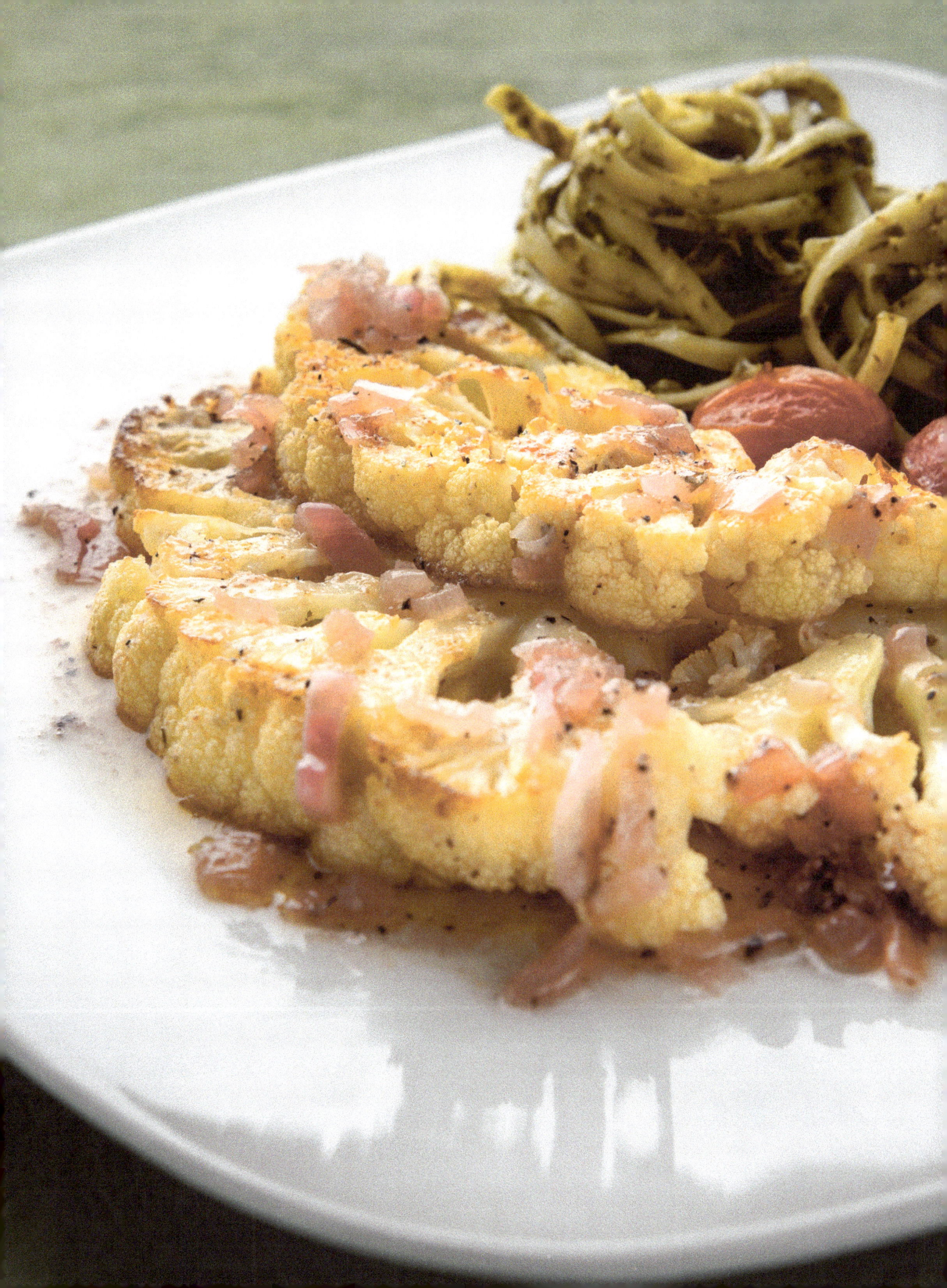

Veggie and Daring Chicken Skewers

Equipment: Deep cookie sheet, outdoor or indoor grill, bamboo skewers, deep dish with lid, tongs, silicone sauce brush or equivalent

½ package of Daring Plant Chicken Tenders Original, defrosted for 30 minutes and chopped into 2-inch chunks

1 cup each of red bell pepper, orange bell pepper, red onion, and zucchini, cut into 2-inch chunks

¾ cup of coconut aminos

Basting sauce of your choice

Optional: fresh pineapple chunks

Sauce

½ cup tomato sauce

1 teaspoon of Worcestershire sauce or gluten-free vegan Worcestershire

4 garlic cloves, crushed

1 tablespoon of molasses

2 tablespoons of agave syrup or maple syrup

½ teaspoon of hot sauce

Coconut oil cooking spray

Directions:

Soak medium-sized bamboo skewers in water while heating your grill. After 10 minutes of soaking and preheating, skewer two veggie pieces and one chicken piece twice; 2 rows are perfect for each skewer then add a third row of veggies on the bottom.

Lay the skewers on a cookie sheet and pour the coconut aminos on them to completely cover. After about 5 minutes, put the skewers on the grill (use coconut oil cooking spray first) on medium-high heat, turning them every 2 minutes. Baste with the sauce—or your sauce of choice—using a silicone brush. Grill for 12 minutes or until slightly charred. Take the skewers off the grill and pour the remaining sauce over them. If you'd like leftover sauce, feel free to double the recipe.

Sauce Directions:

Combine all the sauce ingredients and simmer on low in a small saucepan for 10 minutes; keep on low while making skewers. Feel free to whisk the ingredients to evenly combine. Brush it on the cooked skewers as a glaze.

Serves 4 to 6.

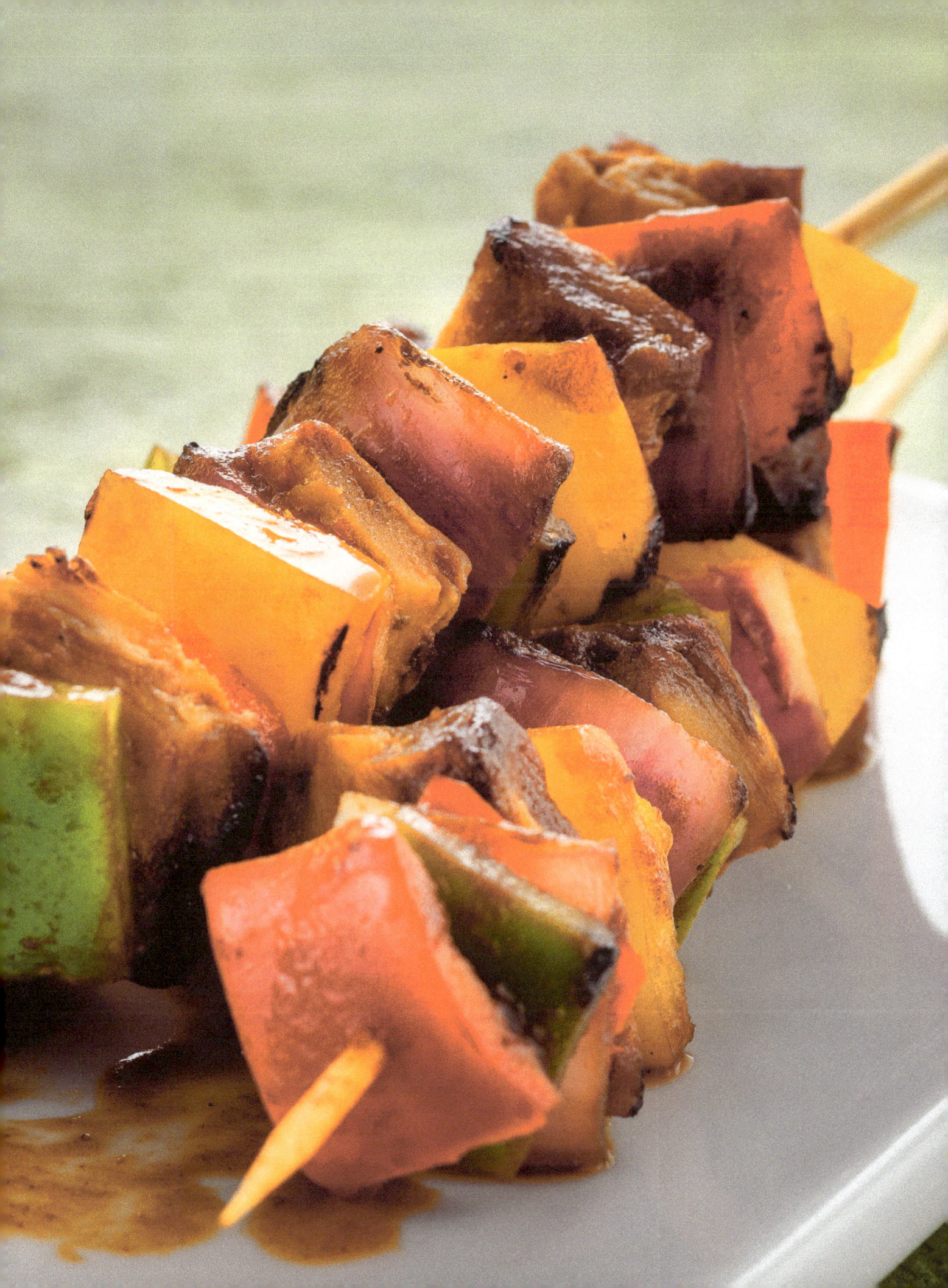

Breakfast Hash

Equipment: 1 large cast iron pan or large, heavy gauge non-stick pan, ice cream scooper

1 tablespoon of extra virgin olive oil

1 medium-sized sweet potato, pre-cooked and cubed

2 small Yukon Gold potatoes, precooked and cubed

1 zucchini, cubed and raw

1 yellow bell pepper, sliced into ½ inch chunks

1 cup broccoli, stalks only, cubed (save florets for another recipe or snack)

2 tablespoons of celery leaves, minced

1 teaspoon of garlic powder

½ teaspoon of salt

½ teaspoon sweet paprika

⅛ teaspoon of ground cinnamon

Fresh parsley sprigs

Directions:

Cook all ingredients by sautéing together to a crispy consistency and sprinkling the seasonings evenly over the mixture while it is cooking. Scoop them out with an ice cream scooper and serve with a side of avocado toast or other toast—preferably Ezekiel bread or a high-fiber, gluten-free substitute if there is an allergy.

Garnish with large sprigs of fresh parsley.

Optional: Add your favorite sauce like organic ketchup or vegan ranch.

Serves 4.

Mushroom Risotto
with Roasted Red Peppers and Sweet Peas

Equipment: Large non-stick frying pan with deep sides, medium cooking pot

2 cups of Arborio rice

2 tablespoons of Miyoko's
    unsalted vegan butter

2 teaspoons of extra virgin olive oil

5 cups of vegetable broth

¾ cup of white wine

2 shallots, finely minced

2 garlic cloves, finely minced

1 cup of cremini mushrooms, sautéed

6 teaspoons of roasted red pepper spread

1 cup of frozen sweet peas, lightly sautéed

½ teaspoon of crushed red pepper

1 teaspoon of Himalayan salt

1 teaspoon of white pepper

6 teaspoons of Follow Your Heart
    Parmesan cheese

Optional: basil leaves and pine nuts

Directions:

Sauté mushrooms in 1 teaspoon of olive oil for approximately 4 minutes, add peas, and sauté for an additional 2 minutes. Set aside.

Preheat a large Dutch oven or a large deep-sided frying pan on the stove for 2 minutes on medium-high heat. In a separate pot, heat the 5 cups of vegetable broth to a low simmer while making the risotto.

Once the Dutch oven is warm, add the butter, the remaining olive oil, and the rice. Stir to completely cover each grain with oil and butter. Keep turning and lightly toasting the rice. Do not brown it. This method should take about 4 to 6 minutes.

Next, add half of the salt and pepper, and the crushed red pepper. Stir for 30 seconds. Add the white wine. Turn up the heat for 3 minutes while the rice simmers and burns off alcohol.

Add the hot broth, one cup every 3 minutes until the rice soaks up most of the liquid while you're constantly stirring and adding the hot broth. Do this for 15 minutes in total. Using up all 5 cups of hot broth, taste the risotto to test the doneness. It should be tender but not soggy and a little al dente with firmness to the rice grains. Feel free to cook for 2 to 4 more minutes until the risotto is perfectly done.

Remove from heat and dish risotto into large plates or pasta bowls. Garnish each serving with one teaspoon of red pepper spread swirled through the center. Add mushrooms to each bowl to one side and sprinkle peas and Parmesan over the top. Serves 6.

Optional: garnish with basil leaves and pine nuts.

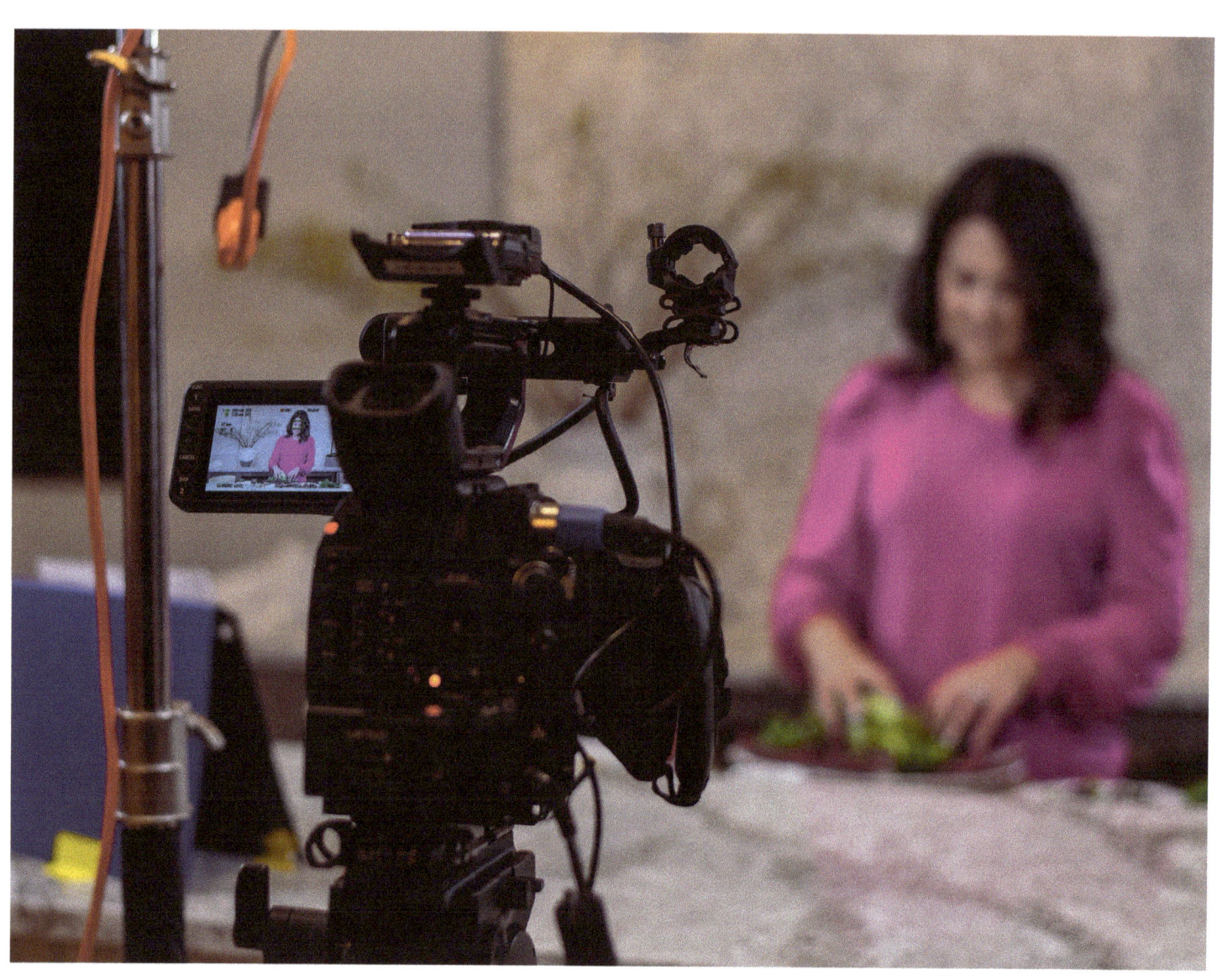

Vegan Crab Cakes

Equipment: Large mixing bowl, cast iron pan, flipping spatula, strainer, paper towels or cloth towel

2 cans of organic whole hearts of palm

1 can of chickpeas, drained

2 tablespoons of nori seaweed flakes

1½ cups of Panko breadcrumbs
   (½ box gluten-free or regular)

1 cup of organic unbleached all-purpose flour
   (gluten-free works too)

6 tablespoons of melted vegan butter

2 tablespoons of Old Bay seasoning

1 teaspoon of dried minced onion

1 teaspoon of black salt that has been turned
   into a powder for even distribution

Directions:

Drain liquid from the hearts of palm, roughly chop, and set aside.

In a separate bowl, lightly mash the chickpeas with a fork so that you don't see the whole bean.

Combine chopped hearts of palm, chickpeas, Panko breadcrumbs, and the rest of the ingredients except the flour and butter.

Make a battering station by lining up your bowl of "crabmeat", a small dish of melted butter, and your shallow dish of flour (feel free to season flour). Form small, 2" x 2" mini crabmeat patties, dip them in the butter, dredge in flour, and fry in oil or feel free to air fry them coated with cooking spray, organic if possible.

Each patty should be fried on medium heat for 3 minutes on each side.

These crab cakes can be reheated in the air fryer or broiled in the oven for 2 to 4 minutes on each side. You can also freeze the crab cakes. If freezing, add two minutes extra to each side on the reheat time.

Makes 12 mini crab cakes. Optional: Enjoy with a vegan mayo or aioli of your choice and finely diced green onions. Feel free to add Old Bay seasoning to your mayo or aioli for a Cajun-flavored sauce. Also, rice or crispy potatoes and a lovely coleslaw would be great sides for this classic dish.

Pro Tip: Put coarse black salt into a small Ziploc and pound with a meat tenderizer until the salt turns into a powder.

Tomato and Spinach JUST Egg Omelet

Equipment: 1 medium non-stick pan, omelet or flipping spatula, cheesecloth

1 cup JUST Egg (liquid vegan egg substitute)

3 tablespoons tomato bruschetta mix in the jar (Trader Joe's) or fresh Roma tomato slices, omitting the seeds

1 cup of sautéed spinach with water squeezed out

½ teaspoon garlic and herb no salt seasoning

¼ teaspoon kosher salt

¼ teaspoon fresh black pepper

⅛ teaspoon cayenne pepper

½ tablespoon of avocado oil

Two slices of vegan Violife Provolone Cheese

Directions:

Sauté fresh baby spinach in a pan until wilted, approximately 3 to 4 minutes. Remove from heat. Gather half of the wilted spinach into a cheesecloth and squeeze out all the liquid, or as much as you can. Repeat with the second half. Lay dry spinach on a cutting board and finely chop.

Heat a saucepan or omelet pan on medium heat and pour in the oil once heated. Poor JUST Egg in the pan and turn the heat down to medium-low. Gently move the JUST Egg around the pan for approximately 5 minutes, but make sure there is a crusty seal at the bottom. Next, add tomatoes and spinach plus seasoning. Gently fold the omelet in half and cover for an additional 2 minutes on low. Finally, put 2 slices of cheese (cut into strips for even distribution) on top of the omelet and put the lid back on for an additional 4 minutes.

Serve with your favorite sides. This omelet will never disappoint and is close to a chicken egg omelet when using the technique above. Each omelet will serve two people by slicing in half or one large omelet for a hearty appetite.

Bonus VIDEO TUTORIAL

 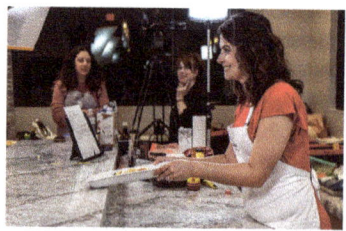

Password: Z1977Fsg1111$

Note: Save the password to your browser for easier access

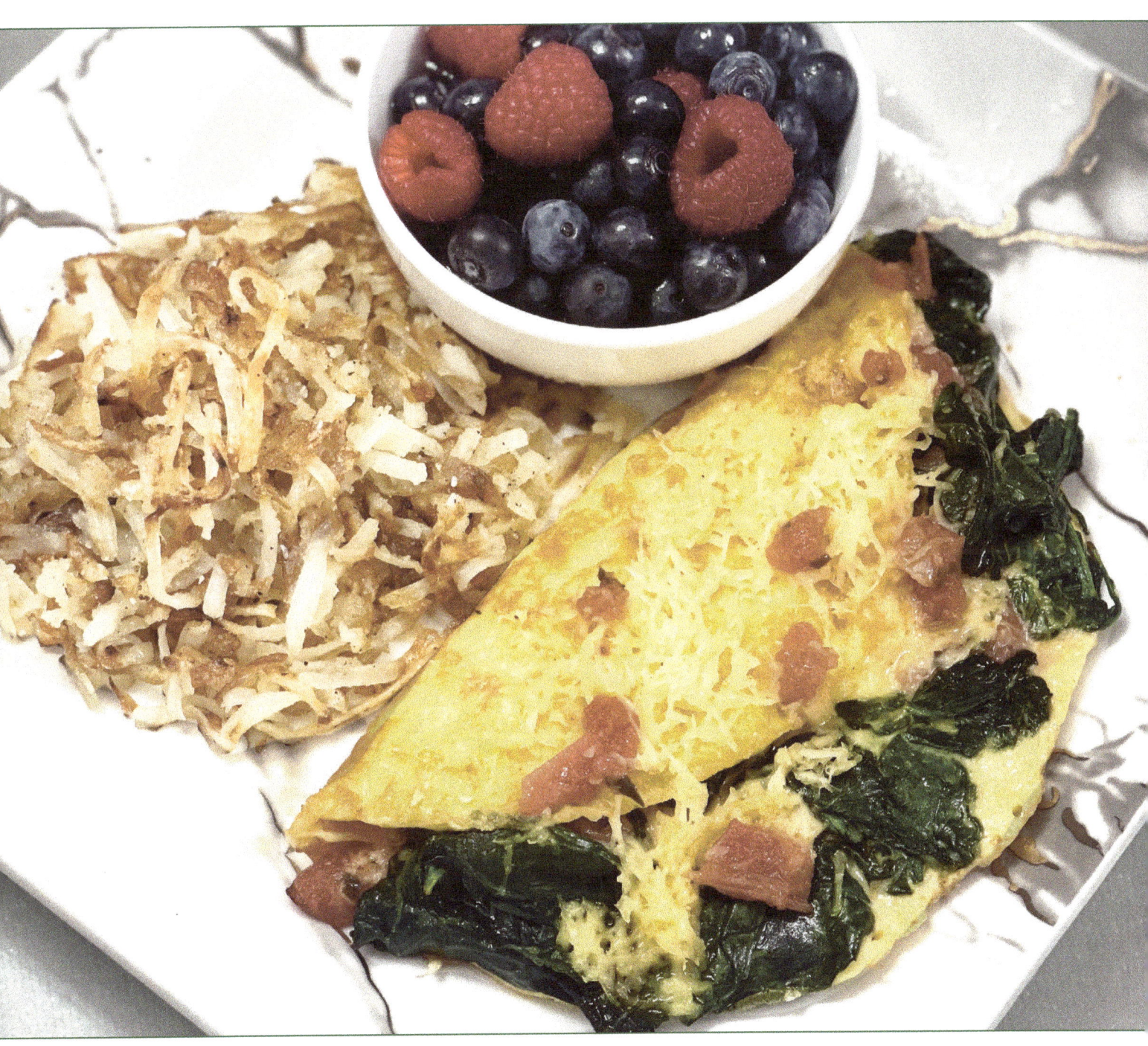

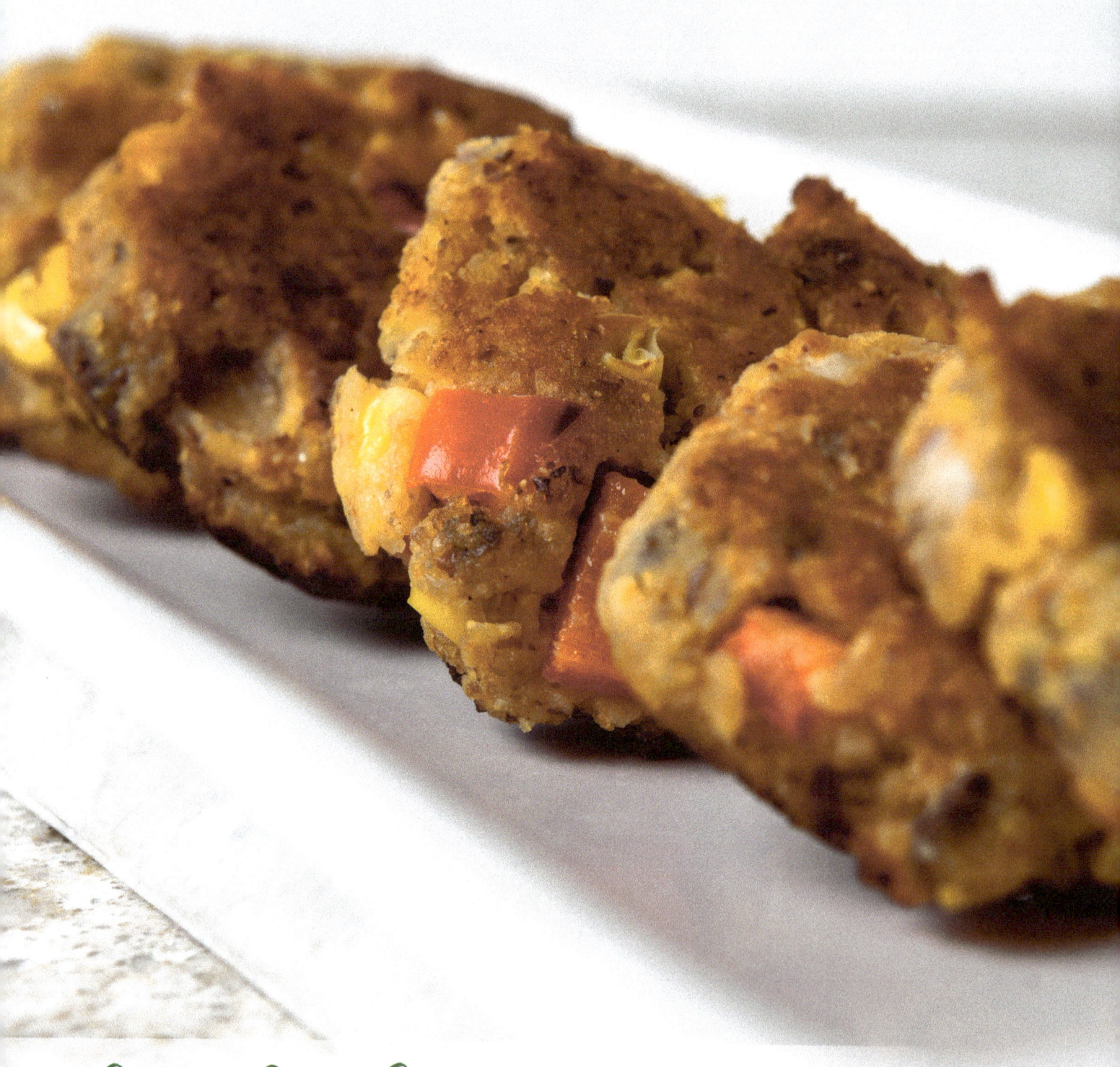

Crispy Corn Griddle Cakes

Recipe and Bonus Video QR Code Pages 74 & 75

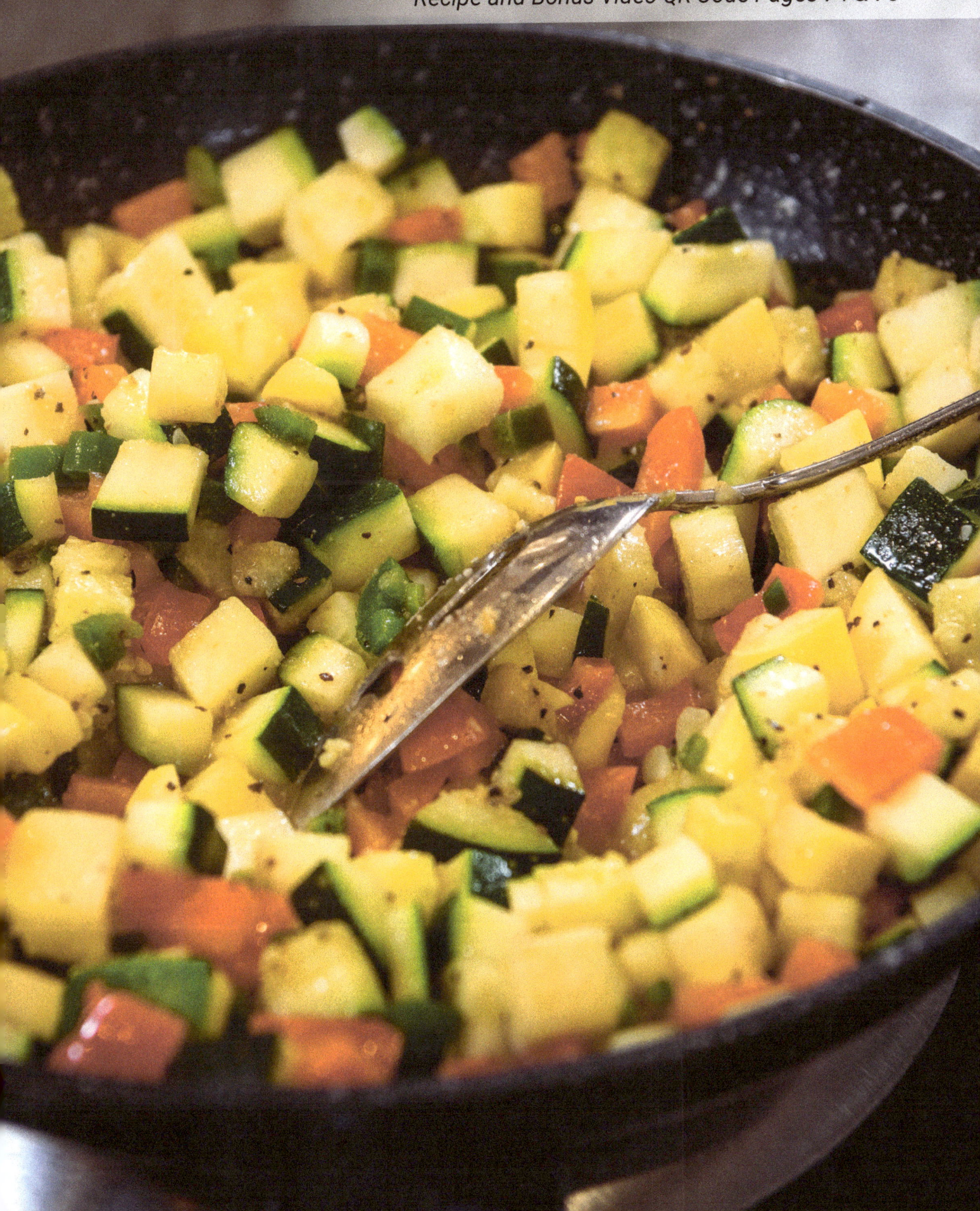

Vegan Shepherd's Pie

Equipment: 9" x 12" baking dish or 8 baking ramekins, potato ricer, large saucepan, large cooking pot, whisk, chef knife

2 cups of ground pea protein or soy curls

5 medium russet potatoes

1 teaspoon of coconut aminos

½ cup of red lentils, halfway cooked

1 small package of frozen mixed vegetables

2 small shallots, finely chopped

4 cloves of garlic, finely minced

2 tablespoons of vegan Worcestershire sauce

2 tablespoons of all-purpose unbleached organic flour or 2 tablespoons of all-purpose gluten-free flour

4 tablespoons of Miyoko's unsalted vegan butter

1 tablespoon of extra virgin olive oil

1 tablespoon of mushroom bouillon

4½ cups of hot vegetable broth

1 teaspoon of Himalayan salt

½ teaspoon of black pepper

¼ teaspoon of crushed red pepper

Extra virgin olive oil cooking spray

Optional: 1 cup of Ian's Original Panko Brea crumbs (gluten-free) mixed with 4 tablespoons of Miyoko's melted butter; combine to form a buttered breadcrumb mixture

Directions:

Peel and chop the potatoes into 2-inch pieces. Boil for 13 minutes on medium-high heat. Drain and spread on a cookie sheet to cool for 5 minutes. Rice the potatoes, a few pieces at a time, with the potato ricer and put them back into the same pan with 2 tablespoons of butter and ½ cup of vegetable broth. Season with half the salt and pepper or to taste. Stir the riced potatoes rapidly with a hand whisk for about 1 minute until you have thoroughly combined the broth and seasonings. Set aside.

In a large saucepan, heat the remaining 2 tablespoons of butter until it's slightly melted. Make a roux by adding the flour while briskly whipping the butter. This should be done on medium-high heat. Add the remaining heated vegetable broth slowly to the roux. Keep whisking slowly until the sauce thickens. Add about ½ cup per minute for a total of 8 minutes. Put on a low simmer for 8 more minutes. Turn off the heat and set aside.

In another large saucepan, add ½ tablespoon of olive oil, shallots, and garlic and sauté on medium heat for about 4 minutes, turning frequently. Next, add the rest of the ingredients, excluding soy curls or pea protein, and 1 tablespoon of vegan Worcestershire sauce. Cook for an additional 6 minutes on a low simmer. Add the roux and vegetable broth mixture to this pan to combine, then set aside. *(continued)*

Take the soy curls or pea protein and sauté them in a saucepan with the other half tablespoon of olive oil. Cook for 4 minutes and add the remaining Worcestershire sauce to this mixture. Cook for another 2 minutes. Add this mixture to the other combined mixture excluding the whipped potatoes.

In the 9" x 12" baking pan, layer the veggie gravy mixture at the bottom of the pan. Add the whipped potatoes as the second layer by spreading them evenly or use a piping bag to make pretty swirls on top. Optional: sprinkle the top with breadcrumbs and butter mixture.

Bake at 375ºF for 25 minutes. Remove from the oven and cool for 10 minutes. Cut into large squares and scoop onto plates or bowls.

Tastes amazing with a side of spring green salad. Serves 6 to 8, depending on your serving size.

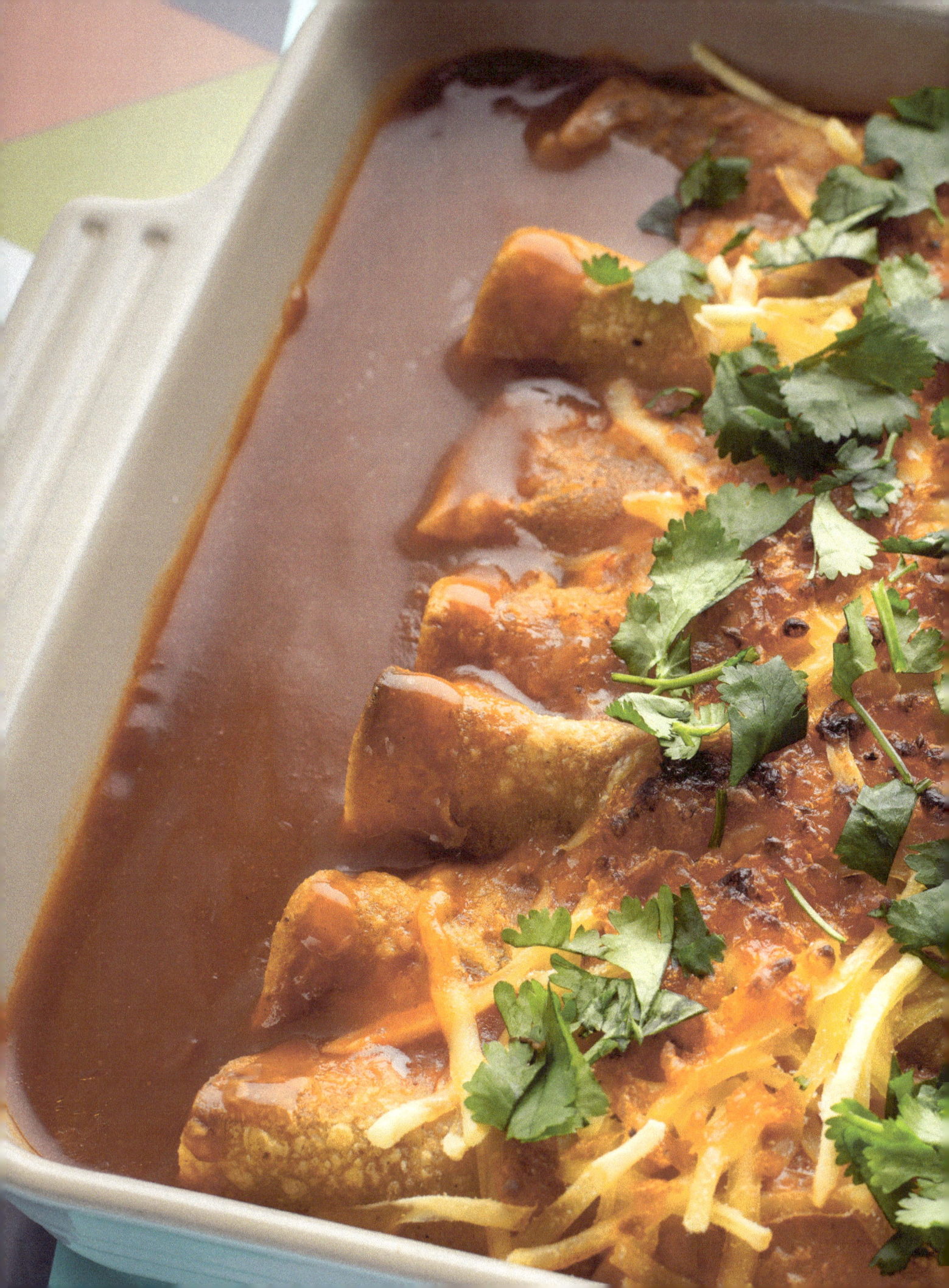

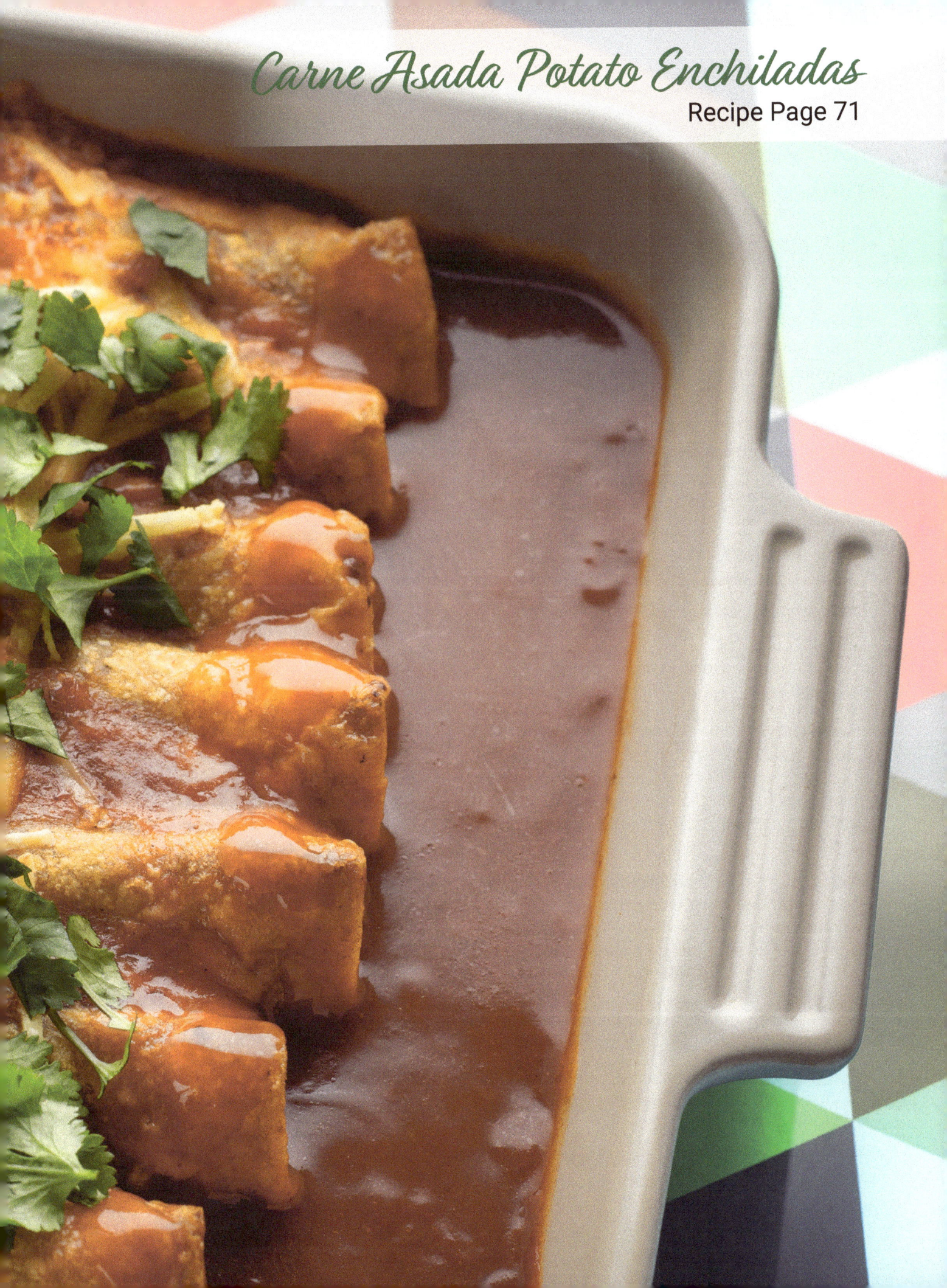

Carne Asada Potato Enchiladas

Recipe Page 71

Carne Asada Potato Enchiladas

Equipment: Large frying pan or sauté pan, small frying pan, large baking dish

- 1 package each of Abbot Butcher Plant-Based "Chorizo" and Ground "Beef"
- 2 small cans of roasted green chiles
- 3 small Yukon yellow potatoes, boiled and smashed with a fork
- 1 zucchini, chopped into ¼-inch cubes and roasted
- 1 small head of cauliflower, chopped and roasted
- 1 package of Chao Creamery Mexican Style Blend Plant-Based Shreds
- ½ tablespoon or more, depending on the number of enchiladas, of Adobe Seasoning
- 1 tablespoon of taco seasoning
- 1 tablespoon of onion powder
- 1 tablespoon of freeze-dried garlic
- 1 teaspoon of garlic salt
- 1 teaspoon of black pepper
- 8 oz. or more of avocado oil for frying
- 30 organic yellow corn tortillas

Directions:

Sauté the chorizo and ground beef in a cast-iron pan with diced green chilies and the rest of the seasoning except the taco seasoning, garlic, salt, and pepper. Sauté for only 5 minutes and set aside.

Roast zucchini and cauliflower, boil potatoes, and assemble in line with carne asada mixture. Fry the corn tortillas and set aside. Each tortilla only takes 20 seconds on each side in a 1-inch bath of avocado oil. Roll each corn tortilla with potato, carne asada, cauliflower, and zucchini. The rest of the seasonings that weren't used for the plant-based meat will go on the cauliflower.

Pour half of the enchilada sauce into a baking dish and add corn tortillas row by row. Top with remaining enchilada sauce.

Next, sprinkle with Chao cheese sparingly. Bake at 375°F for 12 minutes. Serves 6 to 8.

Enchilada Sauce Options
You can purchase already-made enchilada sauce, one 15 oz. can plus one can of tomato sauce, or follow the recipe below.

Homemade Enchilada Sauce

Equipment: Blender, medium pot

- 15 oz. dried chiles, your choice
- 1 chipotle pepper from a can
- 1 15 oz. can of plain tomato sauce
- 3 cloves of garlic, finely minced
- 1 teaspoon of smoked paprika
- 2 teaspoons of ground cumin
- 3 tablespoons of No Chicken bouillon
- 2 cups of hot water
- 3 teaspoons of organic unbleached cane sugar
- Salt to taste

Directions:

1. Prep the dried chiles: Before we can use the chiles, we need to remove the top stem by tearing it off. Then remove most of the seeds by shaking the chiles until they fall out of the opening where the stem was.

2. Reconstitute the chiles: Place the chiles in a large pot, then pour enough water into the pot to cover them. Over medium-low heat, let them simmer for 10 to 20 minutes, or until the chiles turn red and are soft. Reserve both the chiles and the liquid for the next step.

3. Add the tomato sauce, garlic, hot water, and seasonings to a large saucepan. Heat until a low simmer.

4. Purée all ingredients in a blender and simmer on the stove until ready to serve. All ingredients include the above tomato sauce mixture and reconstituted chiles.

Garnish with cilantro sprigs and an optional sauce like vegan avocado crema or plant-based sour cream.

Serves 8 to 10.

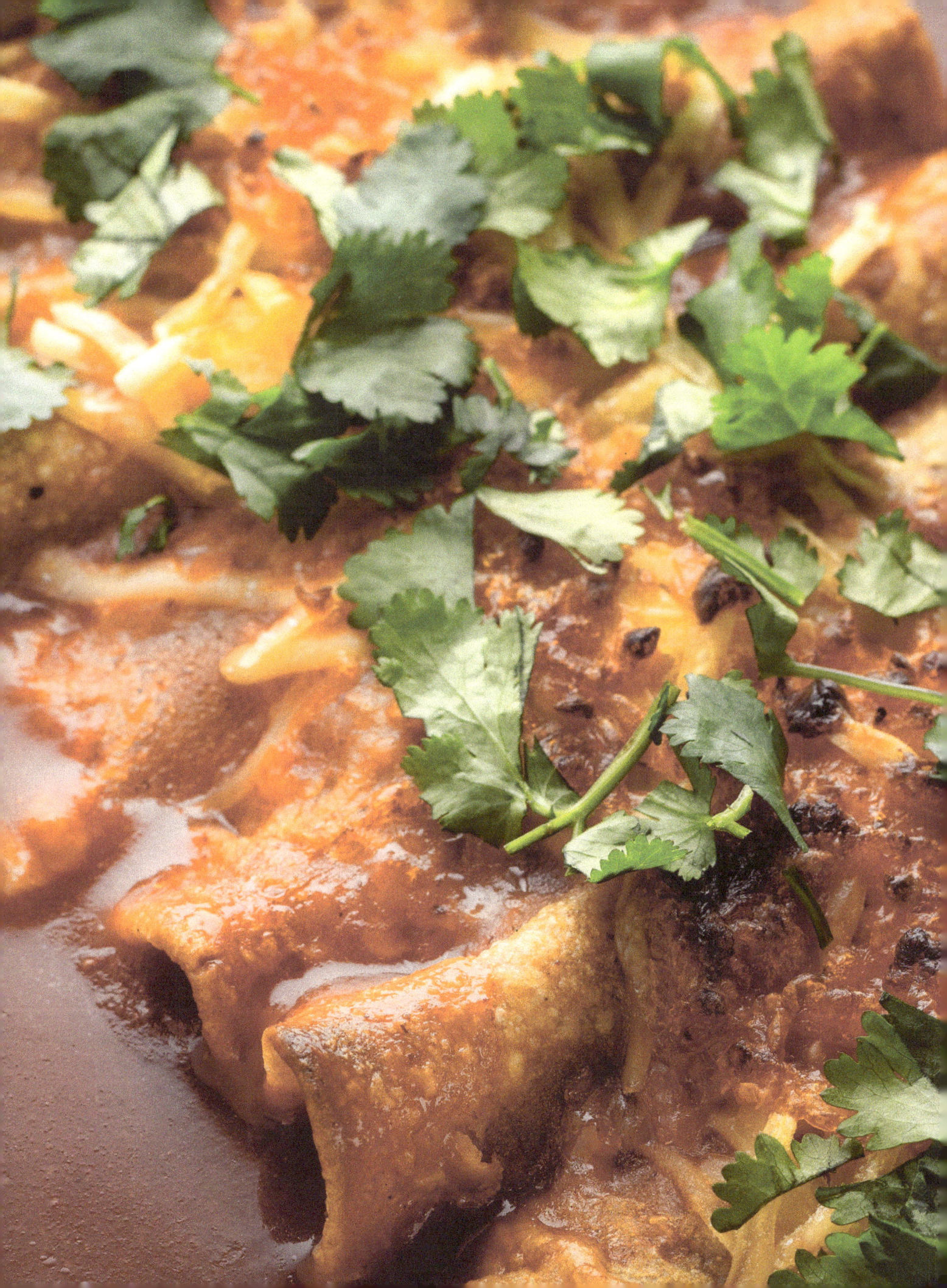

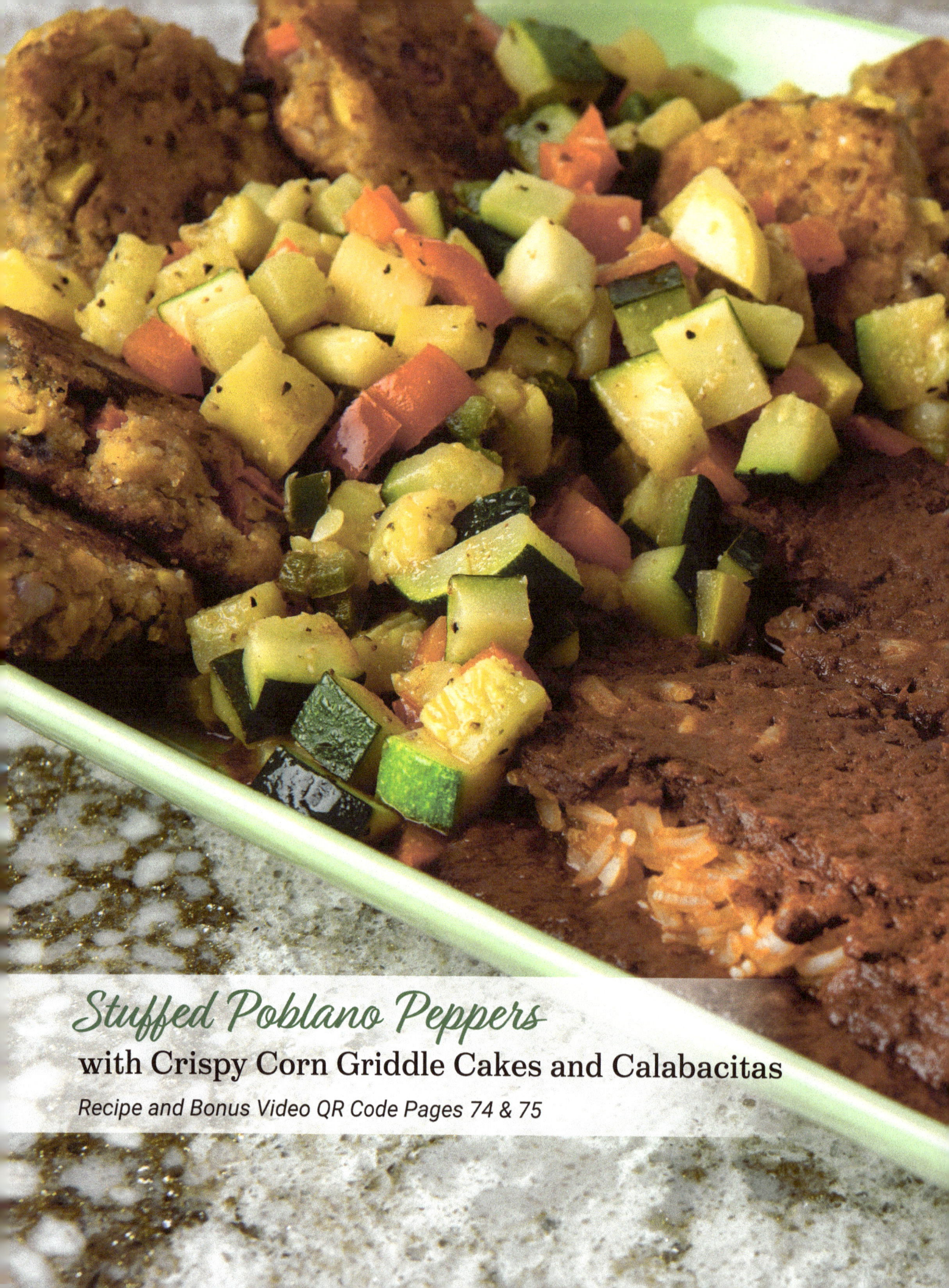

Stuffed Poblano Peppers
with Crispy Corn Griddle Cakes and Calabacitas
Recipe and Bonus Video QR Code Pages 74 & 75

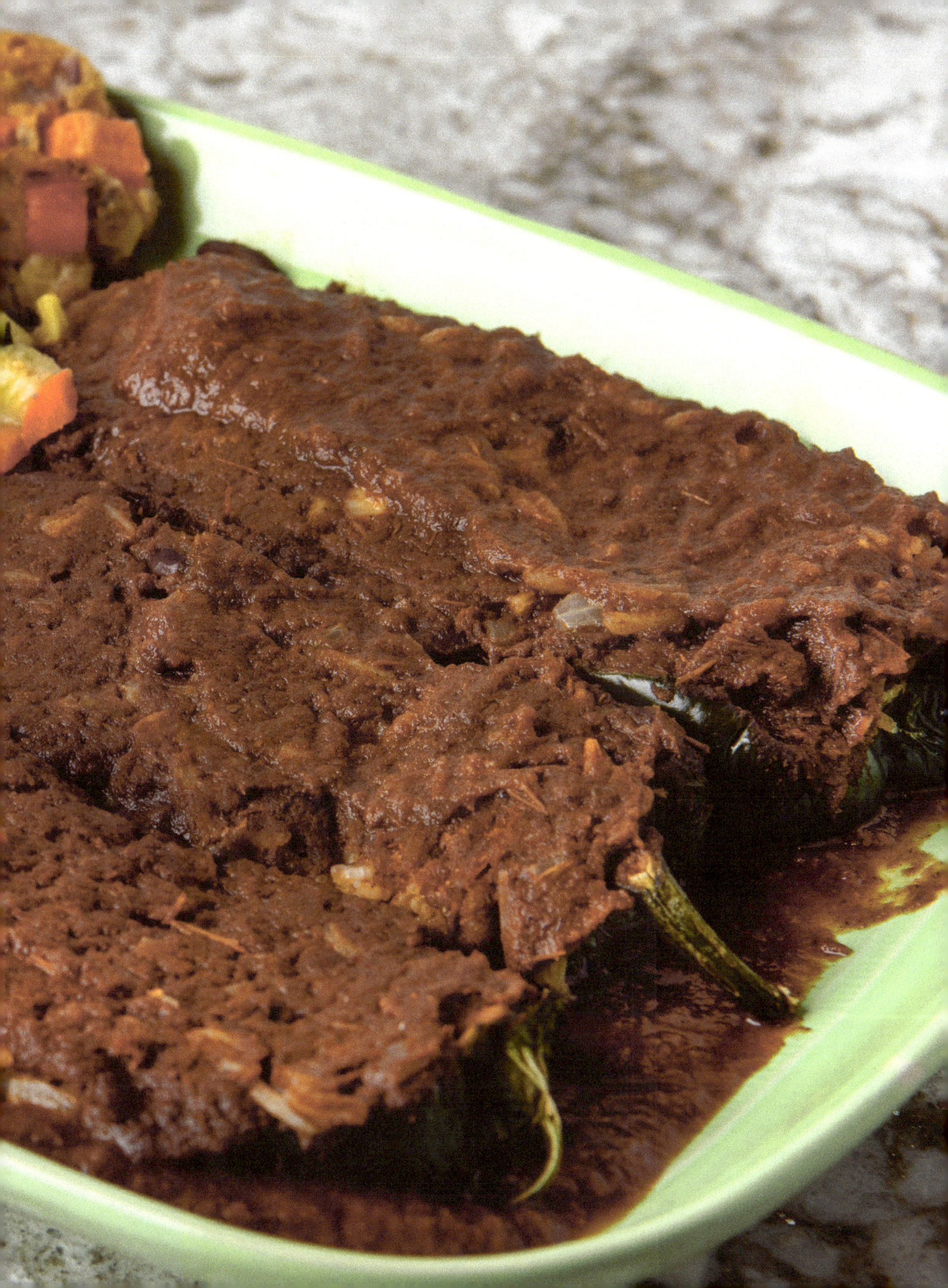

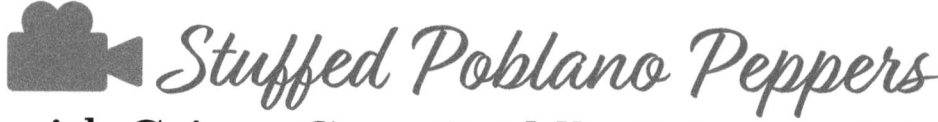

Stuffed Poblano Peppers

with Crispy Corn Griddle Cakes and Calabacitas

Equipment: 2 cookie sheets, medium cooking pot, chef knife

4 large poblano peppers, sliced in half with seeds removed

4 cups of cooked jasmine rice (cook 4 minutes under the cooking time)

1½ cups of black beans, drained (canned or freshly cooked)

1 yellow onion, finely chopped and sautéed for 5 minutes

4 teaspoons of golden raisins

4 tablespoons of ground walnuts

2 small cans of organic enchilada sauce (or from the recipe on page)

Crispy, Sweet Corn Griddle Cakes

Equipment: Large mixing bowl, cast iron pan

Directions on pg 75

½ cup of organic soy milk

½ cup of creamed corn

1 cup of frozen sweet corn, thawed

1 tablespoon of fresh lemon juice

¾ cup of gluten-free all-purpose flour

½ cup of organic sweet potato flour

½ cup of organic yellow cornmeal

1 teaspoon of baking powder

2 flax eggs

½ cup of organic blue corn chips, crushed

1 tablespoon of shallots, minced

1 teaspoon of garlic, minced

¼ cup of red bell pepper, finely chopped

½ teaspoon of cayenne pepper

½ teaspoon of cumin

½ teaspoon of chili powder

¼ cup of agave syrup

¼ cup of avocado oil

1 teaspoon salt

½ teaspoon of black pepper

Directions for the Stuffed Peppers:

Slice poblano peppers in half lengthwise, remove seeds and set aside. Cook rice according to package directions, subtracting 2 minutes from cooking time, promptly removing from heat and placing onto a cookie sheet to cool while you assemble the rest of the rice filling. Sauté the yellow onion in 1 teaspoon of oil for 5 minutes. Add the ground walnuts and sauté for 2 more minutes. Turn off heat and set the pan aside. Add golden raisins to the mixture and let cool for 5 minutes or more.

Heat the canned enchilada sauce (or homemade sauce) in a medium saucepan on a low simmer for 10 minutes. Take cooled rice and bean mixture and stuff each halved pepper with enough mixture to barely fit to the top. Do not overfill. Place rows of halved peppers on a deep-sided cookie sheet. Top each pepper with 2 tablespoons of sauce. Bake at 350°F for 18 minutes. Remove peppers from the oven and serve immediately with corn cakes and calabacitas. Use the remaining sauce by adding a dollop to each plate for dipping during the meal.

Calabacitas

Equipment: Cast iron pan or medium sauté pan, chef knife or any chopping tool

3 cups of raw zucchini, cubed

1 cup of red bell pepper, finely sliced and cubed

2 jalapeño peppers, seeded and chopped finely

1 cup of raw yellow squash, cubed

1 teaspoon of cumin

1 teaspoon of Chile Limón seasoning

1 teaspoon of garlic salt

½ teaspoon black pepper

1½ tablespoons of avocado oil

Bonus VIDEO TUTORIAL

 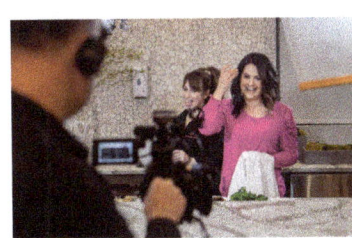

Password: Z1977Fsg1111$

Note: Save the password to your browser for easier access

Directions for Calabacitas:

Prepare all veggies by chopping the zucchini and squash into ½ -inch cubes, finely chopping red pepper and jalapeños, and sprinkling with the remaining seasonings.

Sauté the vegetable mixture for 5 to 7 minutes on medium-high heat. Remove from heat and serve immediately.

Combine corn cakes, calabacitas and stuffed peppers with sauce over the top as a main entrée. This can be a plated meal or a family-style, serve-yourself setup.

Serves 6.

Directions for the Corn Cakes:

Make 2 flax eggs by combining 1 tablespoon of flax meal with 3 tablespoons of warm water for each egg and set aside. Combine the soy milk and the lemon juice and set aside for 5 minutes.

Combine the wet ingredients including the flax eggs and lemon juice/soy milk. Separately, combine all the dry ingredients with a whisk. Add the wet ingredients to the dry ingredients with a whisk, including the corn kernels.

Form the batter into 3-inch patties. Drop 4 patties at a time in hot avocado oil. Cook on medium heat for 7 minutes per side. Lay each patty on a paper towel-lined plate to drain the oil, and lightly salt. Serve alongside your favorite meal. With this meal, serve with calabacitas and stuffed peppers.

Makes 18 patties.

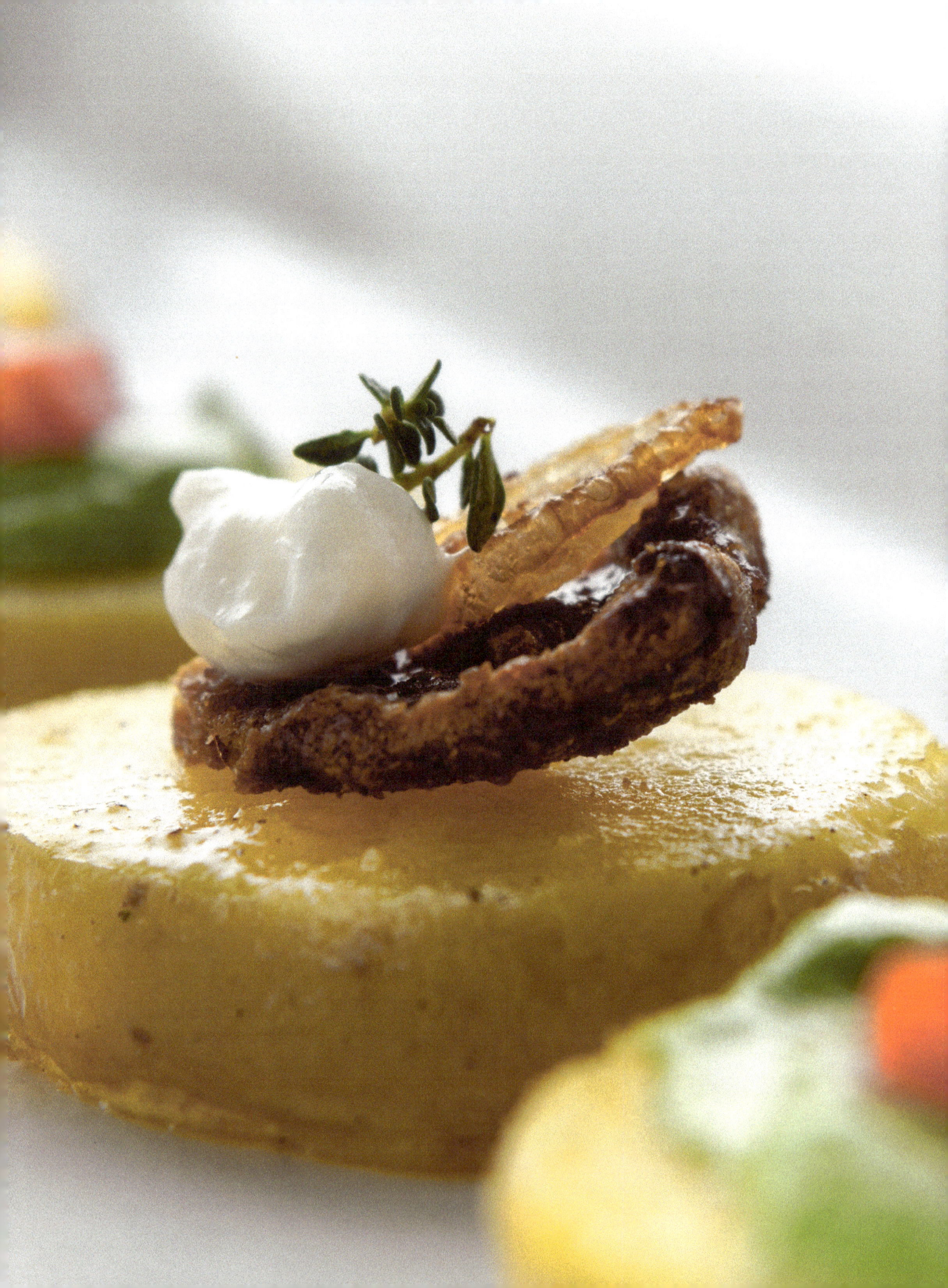

The Perfect Potato

Miso Mashed Potatoes

Greek Cold Garlic Potato Dip

Steak and Yukon Gold Potato Bites

Pesto Potato Poppers

Featured Opposite Page:

Steak and Yukon Gold Potato Bites

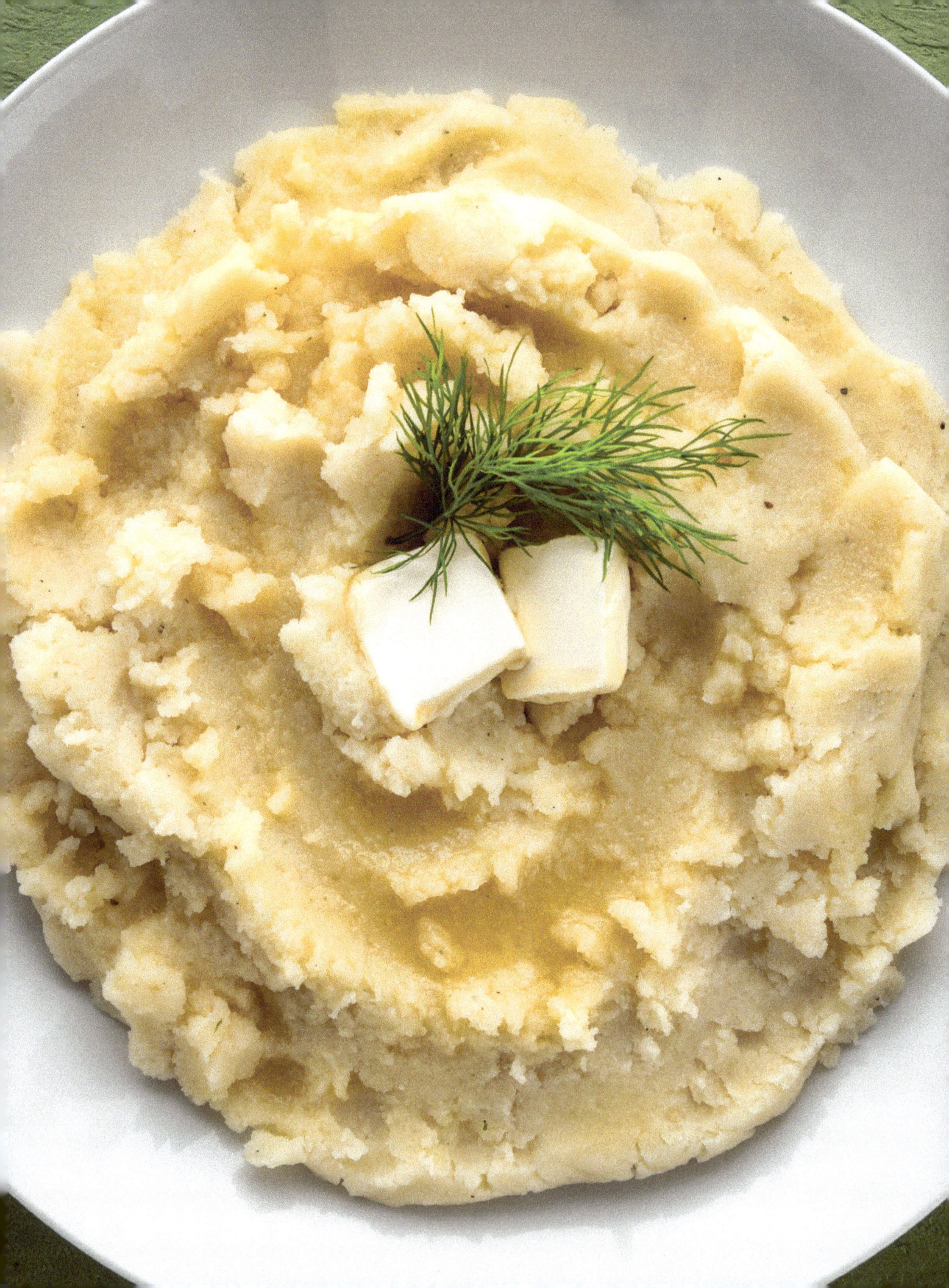

Miso Mashed Potatoes

Equipment: Large cooking pot, potato ricer, cookie sheet, whisk

6–7 russet potatoes, washed, peeled, and cut into 2-inch pieces

4 tablespoons vegan butter

4 cloves of garlic, roasted

1 tablespoon of extra virgin olive oil

1¼ cups of miso broth

(Optional: substitute 1 tablespoon of yellow miso paste dissolved in 1½ cups of hot vegetable broth)

2 tablespoons of Himalayan pink salt

1 teaspoon of white pepper

¼ teaspoon of cayenne pepper

Directions:

Boil chopped potatoes in 6 or more cups of water for 10 minutes. Check potatoes with a fork to determine their doneness. Maybe add 4 or 5 minutes of slow simmering to cook through. Do not overcook. Drain potatoes. Toss the cooked potatoes onto a cookie sheet to dry and partly cool, around 5 minutes.

On a low simmer, heat and whisk the remaining ingredients, except the salt, pepper, and cayenne. Keep on a low simmer until the potatoes are riced.

Immediately rice the potatoes into the same pot you cooked them in and set on the stove at a very low temperature.

Add salt, pepper, and cayenne to riced potatoes, then add hot liquid and whisk until fluffy. Taste the potatoes. What do they need? Salt, more miso? More pepper? Adjust seasonings accordingly.

Serves 4 to 6.

Greek Cold Garlic Potato Dip

Equipment: Potato ricer, small serving bowl

- 4–5 medium russet potatoes
- 2 tablespoons of lemon juice, freshly squeezed
- 2 drops of Young Living Lemon Vitality essential oil, or any food-grade lemon essential oil of your choice
- 6 cloves of garlic, roasted
- ⅛ teaspoon of cayenne pepper
- 2 tablespoons of extra virgin olive oil
- Optional: 1 tablespoon of parsley, minced

Directions:

Peel and chop potatoes into 1-inch chunks. Boil on a low simmer in 6 cups of water for 12 minutes. Drain and cool the potatoes on a cookie sheet for 5 minutes, no more. Put chunks into a potato ricer and rice all the potatoes into a medium mixing bowl. Set aside.

Combine all the remaining ingredients, except parsley and 1 tablespoon of olive oil, by blending them in a small blender cup. Whisk all the blended ingredients into the riced potatoes until you achieve a fluffy dip (not a mashed potato, this is more of a fluffy dip consistency).

Transfer potato dip to a serving bowl, drizzle with remaining olive oil in a spiral design, and sprinkle with minced parsley. Serve with pita chips or your dipper of choice. Serve as an appetizer for 4 to 6.

Roasted Garlic

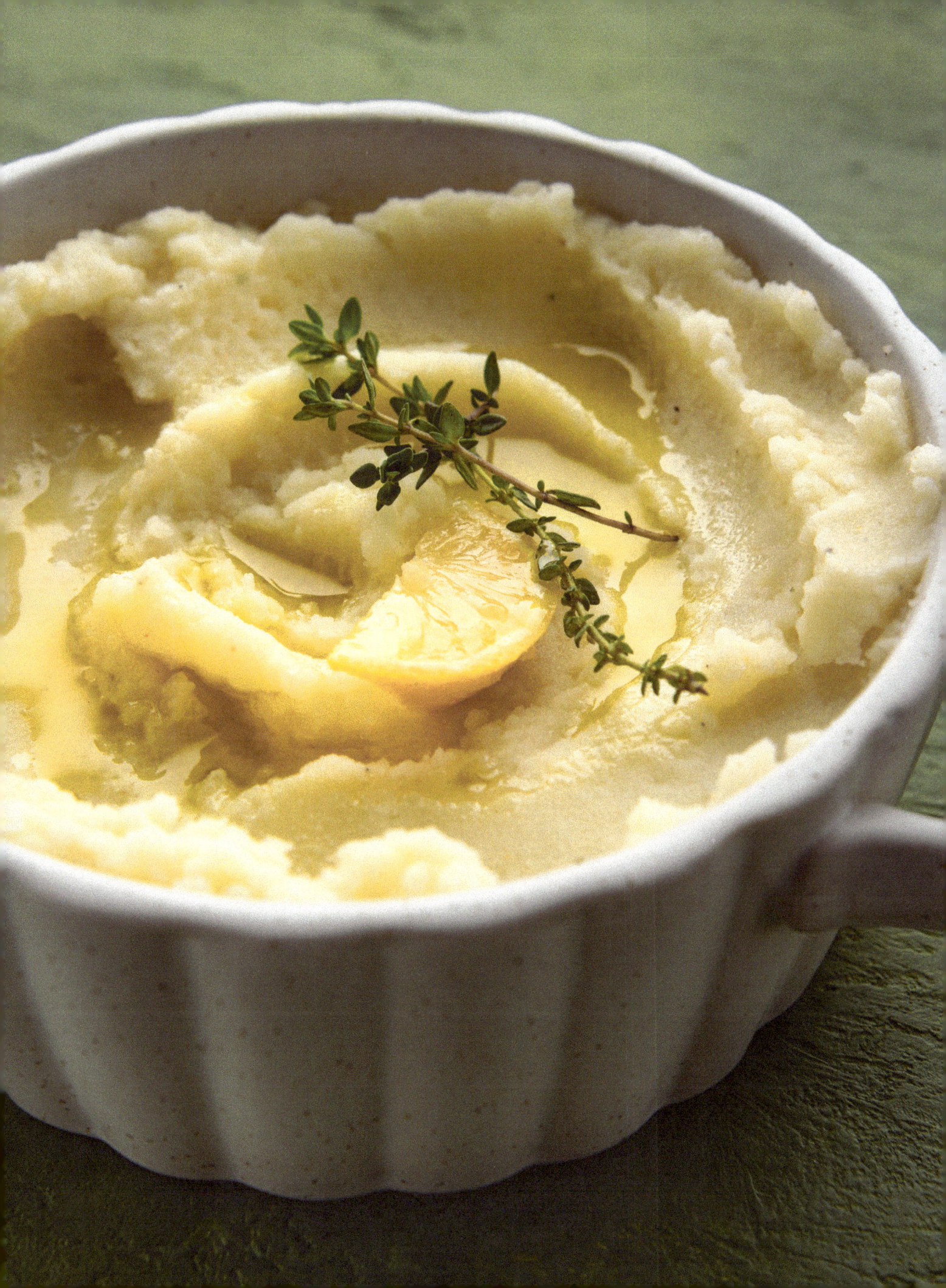

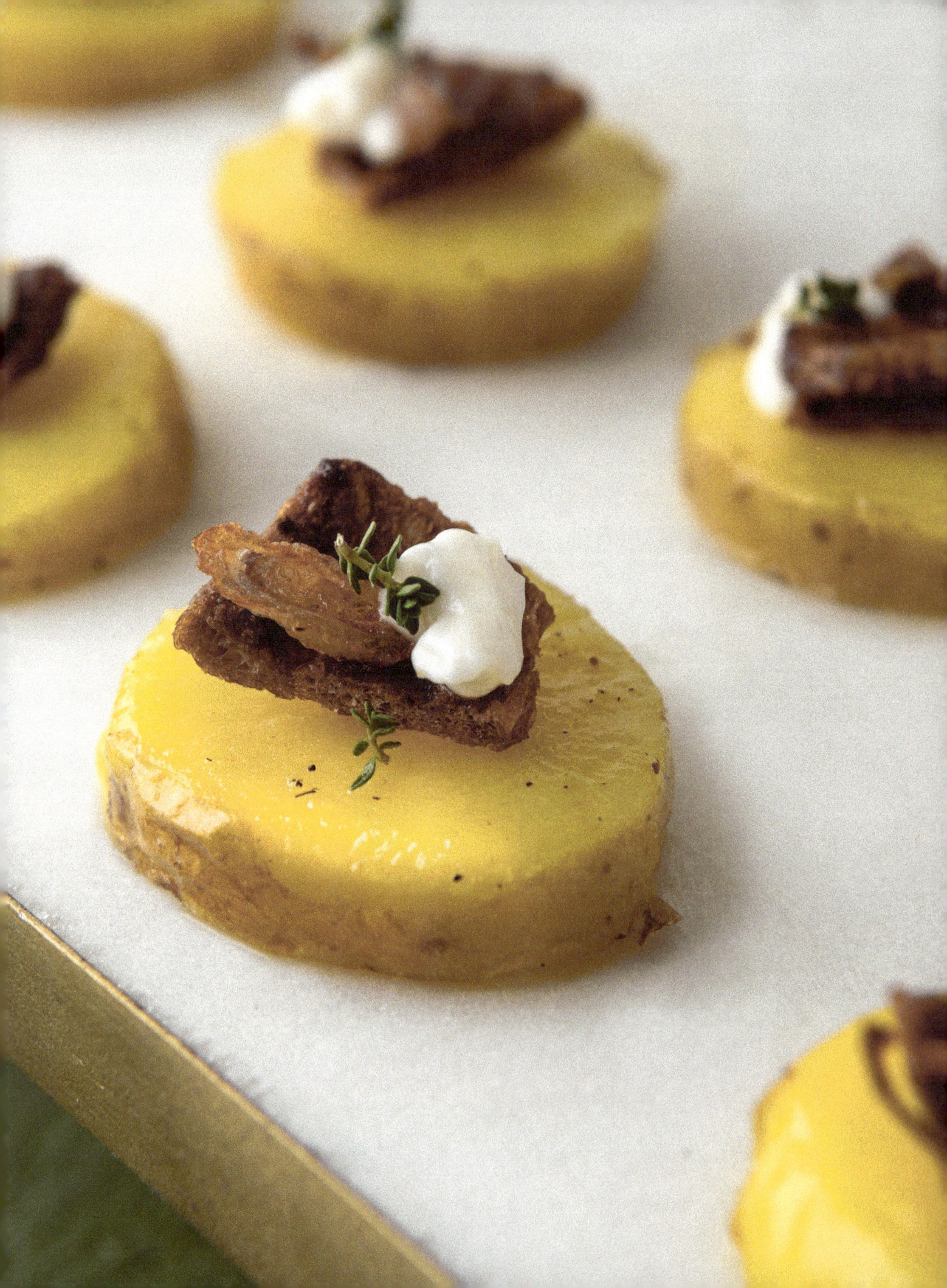

Steak and Yukon Gold Potato Bites

Equipment: Large cooking pot,
2 cookie sheets

10 small Yukon Gold potatoes

12 non-GMO textured soy protein strips or
   Gardein beefless tips,
   or gluten-free equivalent

2 tablespoons of vegan Worcestershire sauce
   or vegan, gluten-free Worcestershire sauce
   from savoryspiceshop.com

2 tablespoons of vegan mayo

1½ tablespoons of extra virgin olive oil

4 sprigs of fresh thyme

1 teaspoon of garlic salt

1 teaspoon of black pepper

Optional: ½ cup of finely chopped and
   cooked portobello mushrooms

Directions:

Boil whole potatoes for 11 minutes. Remove from heat and cool. Rehydrate soy by covering the strips with 1 cup of boiling water for 5 minutes. Drain and cool.

Slice potatoes into ½-inch thick coins and set aside. Evenly add 1 tablespoon of the Worcestershire sauce to the strips. Assemble the potato coins onto two cookie sheets or baking dishes with ½ soy strip on top of the coin until you get 24 bites. Drizzle olive oil on top, attempting to not get too much oil on the soy strips. Liberally sprinkle with garlic salt and pepper. Bake at 425°F for 7 minutes, then remove from oven. Remove thyme leaves from stems and sprinkle over the bites.

Combine the remaining Worcestershire sauce, cooked and cooled mushrooms, and mayo with a whisk. With a very small spoon or Ziploc bag with the corner cut out, dollop the mushroom mayo on top of each bite. Serves 8 for appetizers.

Pesto Potato Poppers

Equipment: Cookie sheet(s), chef knife, blender or blender cup

8 small Yukon Gold potatoes

1 teaspoon of garlic salt

1 teaspoon of black pepper

2 roasted red peppers or 24 roasted red pepper strips

2 tablespoons of extra virgin olive oil

½ cup of vegan mayo

¼ cup of basil leaves, roughly chopped

4 garlic cloves, roasted

¼ cup of pine nuts

1 teaspoon of nutritional yeast

1 teaspoon of balsamic glaze

Directions:

Boil the potatoes in a large pot for 10 minutes. Remove from heat, drain, and cool for 10 minutes. Once cooled, slice them into 1½-inch coins. Try for a uniform size for a prettier appetizer. Lay the coins (24 to 30) on a cookie sheet or two and drizzle them lightly with olive oil. Sprinkle them with half of the garlic salt and pepper. Broil the potatoes in the oven for 6 minutes, then cool them until they are at room temperature.

Meanwhile, combine all the remaining ingredients except the red peppers, remaining garlic salt, and pepper. Blend them in a blender cup to make the creamy pesto topping. Put the pesto topping in the fridge to stay cold.

Slice the red pepper into ½-inch rounds or strips. Set aside.

Assemble the potato poppers by taking each coin and topping it with a teaspoon size dollop of pesto mayo, and a slice of red pepper. The colors will be bright green and red—great for a holiday appetizer!

The recipe makes a minimum of 24 poppers.

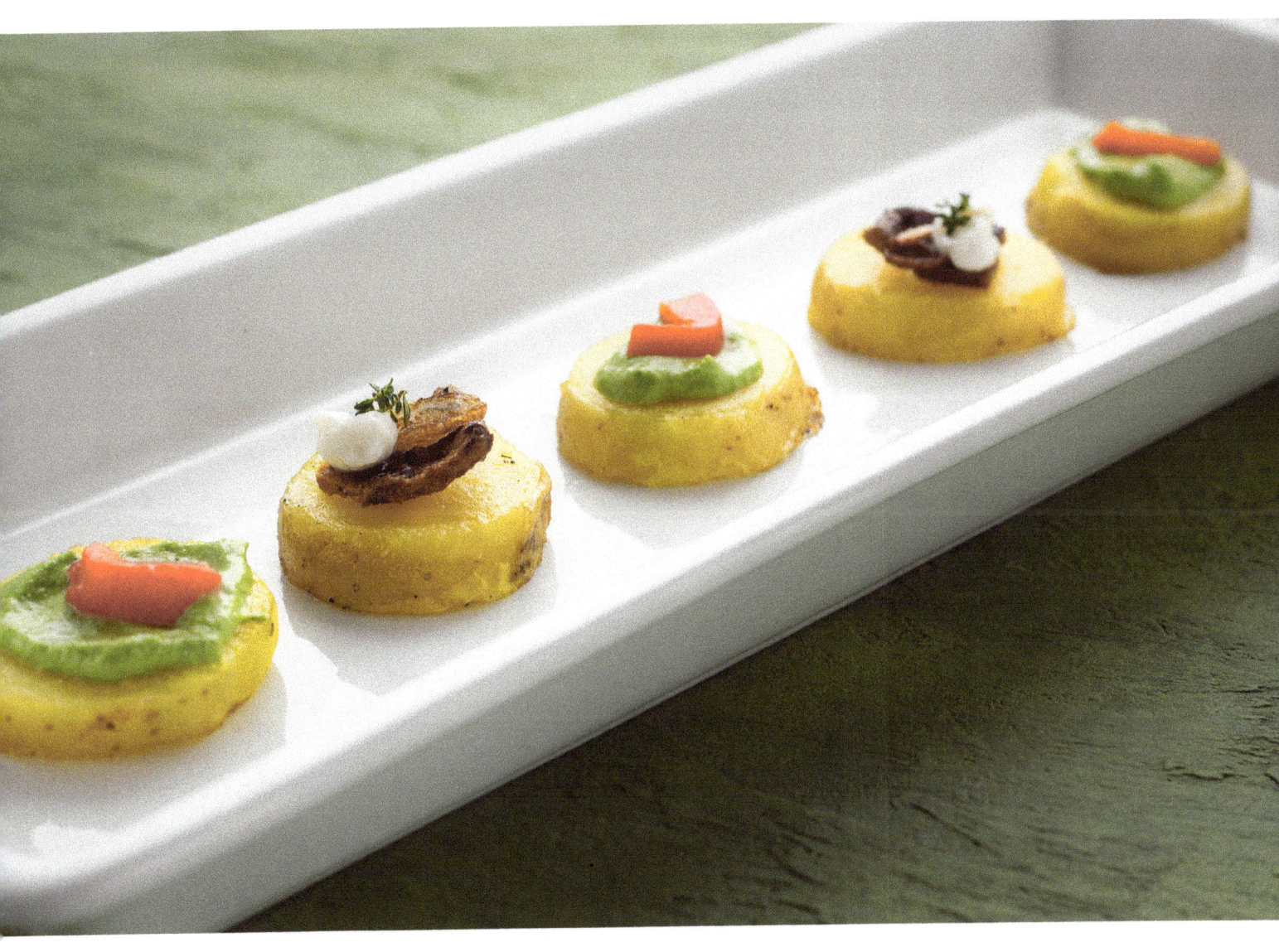

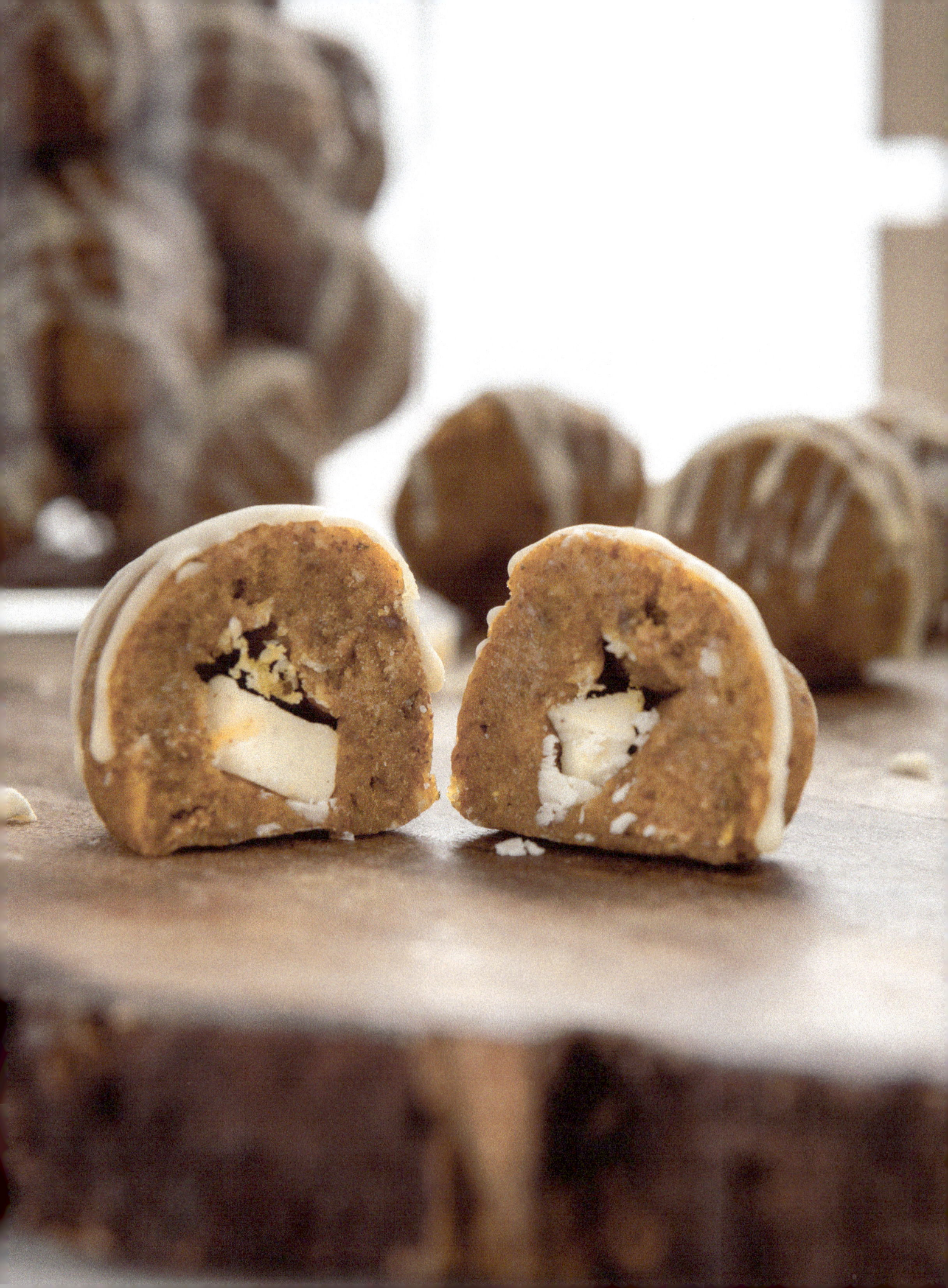

Sweet Things

Wild Blueberry Zucchini Bread with Vegan Cream Cheese Icing

Vegan Bread Pudding

Sticky Rice Pudding with Mango Purée and Coconut Chips

Forest Berry Mousse

Raw Pumpkin Power Bites with White Chocolate Icing

Featured Opposite Page:

Raw Pumpkin Power Bites with White Chocolate Icing

Wild Blueberry Zucchini Bread
with Vegan Cream Cheese Icing

Equipment: Stainless steel or another loaf pan, large mixing bowl, medium mixing bowl, small bowl, cheesecloth, whisk, spatula, measuring cups and spoons, parchment paper

1½ cups organic all-purpose unbleached flour*

½ cup organic unbleached cane sugar

½ cup of monk fruit sugar

1 flax egg (1 tablespoon of flax meal with 3 tablespoons of warm water)

¾ cup unsweetened applesauce

1 tablespoon of molasses

1 teaspoon of baking soda

2 teaspoons baking powder

1 teaspoon of cinnamon

¼ teaspoon nutmeg, freshly grated

1 teaspoon of kosher salt

½ cup coconut oil, melted

2 teaspoons of vanilla bean paste

1 drop of Young Living Cardamon essential oil, or ⅛ teaspoon of cardamom

1½ cups of finely grated zucchini with water squeezed out (cheesecloth)

½ cup dried wild blueberries covered in ¼ cup of organic flour*

¼ cup dried wild blueberries for garnish (Trader Joe's Wild Blueberries for example)

Coconut oil cooking spray

Directions:

Preheat oven to 350°F.

Make the flax egg by adding 1 tablespoon of flax meal to 3 tablespoons of warm water, whisk, and set aside. Combine all wet ingredients (including sugar and monk fruit sugar) except flax egg and grated zucchini. Combine all dry ingredients except blueberries and put in a medium-sized bowl, set aside. Take grated zucchini and divide it in half. Put half of the grated zucchini into the cheesecloth and squeeze out as much of the liquid as you can. Repeat with the other half of the zucchini. Add drained zucchini to wet ingredients and whisk to combine. Add the flax egg to the wet ingredients and whisk to combine. The wet ingredients should be in the large mixing bowl.

Slowly add the combined dry ingredients to the large mixing bowl of wet ingredients. Do not whisk the combined ingredient mixture for more than 2 minutes, no more than 4 minutes for gluten-free.

*You can substitute gluten-free all-purpose flour, 1:1 ratio.

Finally, add the flour-covered blueberries to the batter slowly with a spatula. Pour the entire batter into a parchment-lined loaf pan sprayed with coconut oil cooking spray. Bake for 55 minutes. Remove from oven; check doneness by inserting a toothpick into the middle of the loaf. If it comes out clean with no batter on the toothpick, it's done, if it comes out with batter on it, put it back in the oven for 5 to 7 additional minutes.

Remove the loaf pan from the oven and cool for at least 20 minutes before removing the loaf from the pan. Add icing before serving.

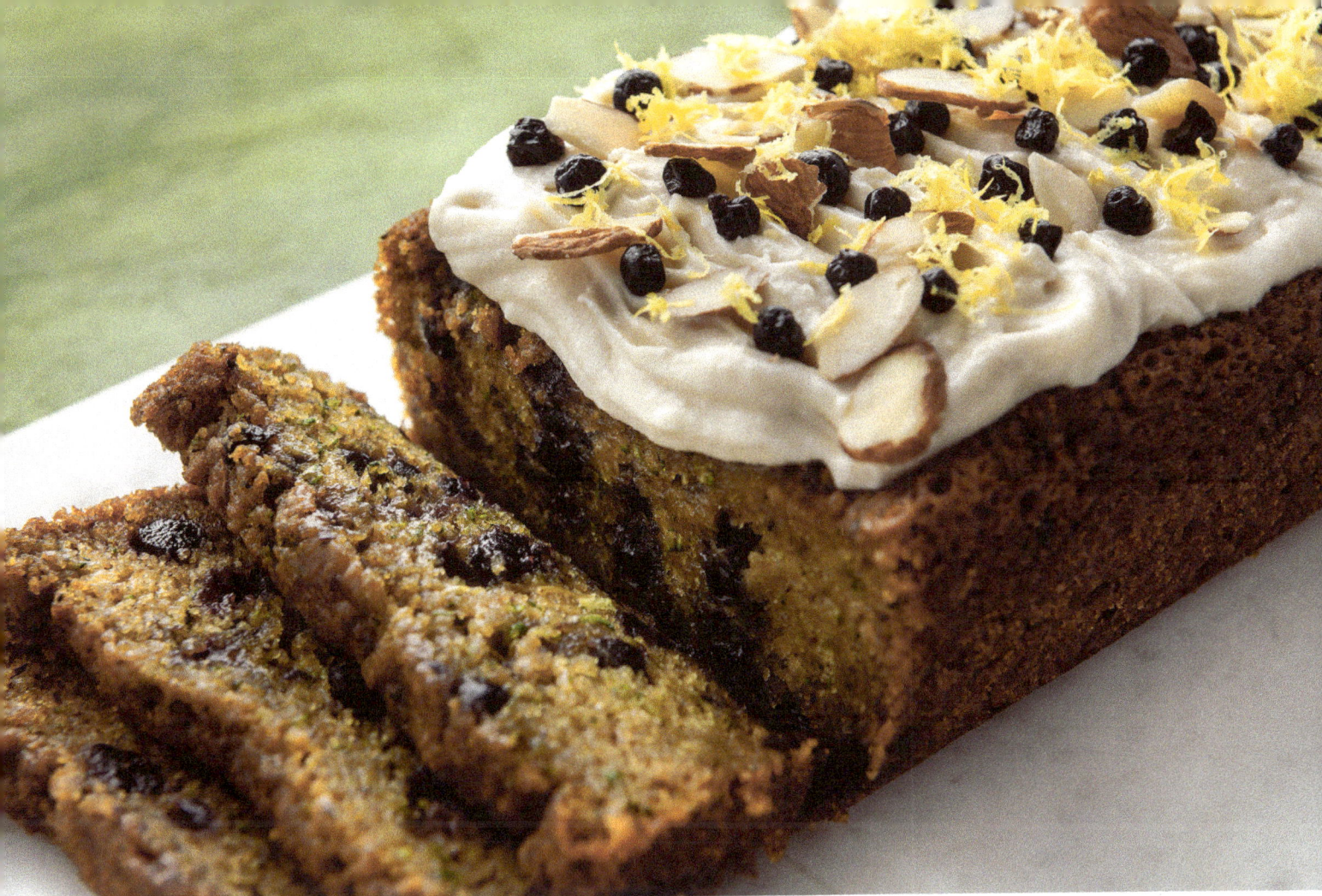

Vegan Cream Cheese Icing

Equipment: Stainless medium-sized mixing bowl, hand mixer with a whisk attachment

1 container of Trader Joe's Vegan Cream Cheese

4 tablespoons of unsalted Miyoko's vegan butter

1½ cups of organic powdered sugar

2 tablespoons of maple syrup

½ teaspoon of kosher salt

1 teaspoon of real almond extract

2 drops of Young Living Lemon Vitality essential oil, or food-grade lemon essential oil of your choice

Garnish with sliced almonds, lemon zest, and a few wild blueberries

Icing Directions:

Soften the cream cheese for at least 30 minutes by letting it sit on the counter at room temperature. Add the measured cream cheese to a cold bowl. Add cold vegan butter to the cold bowl. Add the maple syrup, lemon oil, almond extract, kosher salt, and ½ of the powdered sugar to the cold bowl. Immediately mix slowly with the whisk attachment of a hand mixer until combined, about 2 minutes. Add the remaining powdered sugar and whisk for another 2 minutes.

Scrape the ingredients with a spatula into a large Ziploc bag or use a pastry bag. Press the air out of the Ziploc bag to make sure only the loose icing is remaining in the bag. Refrigerate the icing for at least 30 minutes before adding it to the top of the zucchini bread. Make sure the zucchini bread is cooled before adding the icing. Slice a large corner from the Ziploc bag and squeeze in a zig-zag pattern over the top of the loaf. Garnish with sliced almonds and remaining blueberries.

Serves 8.

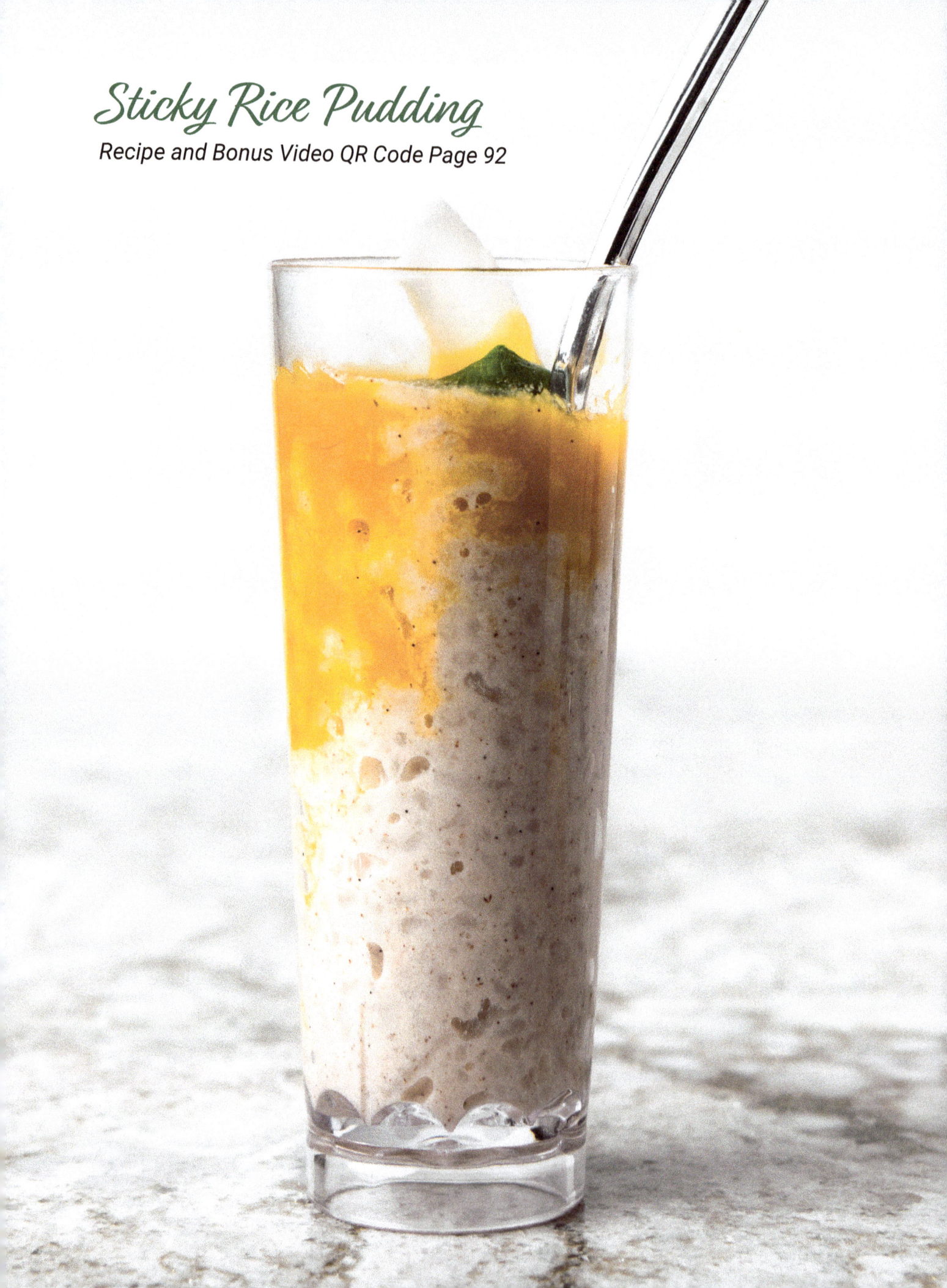

Sticky Rice Pudding

Recipe and Bonus Video QR Code Page 92

Vegan Bread Pudding

Equipment: 8" x 8" baking dish, mixing bowl, whisk

- 4–5 day old or leftover vegan croissants, chopped; feel free to use a gluten-free substitute
- 1 cup of plant milk (preferably soy or macadamia)
- 2 flax eggs (2 tablespoons ground flax meal mixed with 6 tablespoons of warm water, let sit for 5 minutes)
- 2 tablespoons of almond French vanilla coffee creamer
- ¼ cup of organic brown sugar
- ¼ cup of Miyoko's vegan butter
- 2 tablespoons of bourbon vanilla bean paste
- ½ teaspoon of cinnamon
- ½ teaspoon of fresh nutmeg, grated
- 1 5 oz. can of coconut crème (sweeten with ½ cup of organic powdered sugar)

Directions:

Whisk the ingredients briskly, except the butter and croissants, in a medium mixing bowl.

Pour the whisked mixture over the chopped croissants inside a 8" x 8" pan that has been sprayed with cooking spray of your choice. Chop butter into small chunks and sprinkle evenly over the mixture.

Bake at 400°F for 20 minutes. Turn off the oven and let sit inside for 10 minutes. Remove from oven and portion into 1 cup serving sizes. Drizzle with whipped and sweetened coconut crème.

Serves 6.

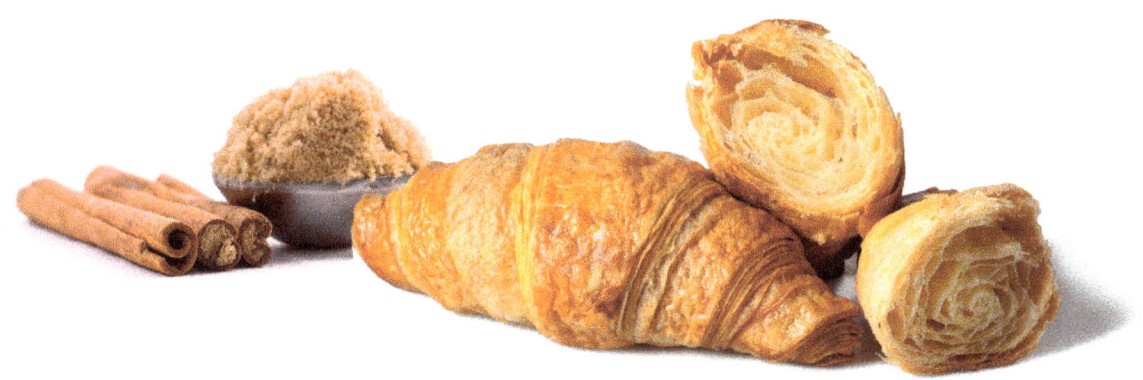

Sticky Rice Pudding
with Mango Purée and Coconut Chips

Equipment: Rice cooker or medium pot, large mixing bowl, medium mixing bowl, spatula, mini serving bowls

4 ⅔ cups of sticky rice cooked and cooled, use organic premium short grain or sushi rice; rice should be sticky and slightly dry (2 cups of dry rice with 2½ cups of water, cook for 15 minutes or according to package directions)

2 cups of unsweetened almond milk

1 cup of full-fat organic coconut milk

¼ cup monk fruit sugar

¼ cup organic unbleached cane sugar

1 teaspoon of cinnamon

¼ teaspoon freshly grated nutmeg

½ teaspoon of kosher salt

2 drops of Young Living Lime Vitality essential oil, or any food-grade lime essential oil of your choice

½ teaspoon of almond bakery emulsion (similar to almond extract) or just use almond extract

2 teaspoons of vanilla bean paste

1½ cups of mango purée from a can (refrigerated)

Chopped mango, thawed from frozen or fresh

Coconut chips

Mint sprigs

Optional: fresh blackberries

Directions:

After cooking and cooling short grain rice, set aside in a large mixing bowl. In a separate medium-sized bowl, combine all wet ingredients and seasonings with a whisk.

Add the wet ingredients and seasonings to the rice and stir well to combine. Do not add the chopped mango, mango puree, coconut chips, mint sprigs, or blackberries. Taste the mixture to determine if it needs more liquid, salt, sugar, or cinnamon.

Refrigerate pudding in a large bowl without mango, mango puree, coconut chips, mint sprigs, or blackberries for one hour or overnight. Serve by adding pudding to mini-serving bowls or appetizer mini-bowls. Garnish with a small teaspoon of mango puree, chopped mango, a coconut chip, mint sprig, and a fresh blackberry.

Serves 6 to 12 depending on the size of the mini bowls.

Bonus VIDEO TUTORIAL

 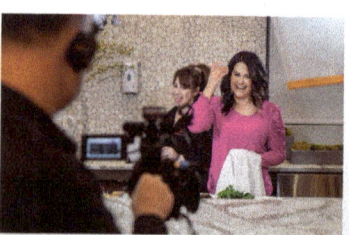

Password: Z1977Fsg1111$
Note: Save the password to your browser for easier access

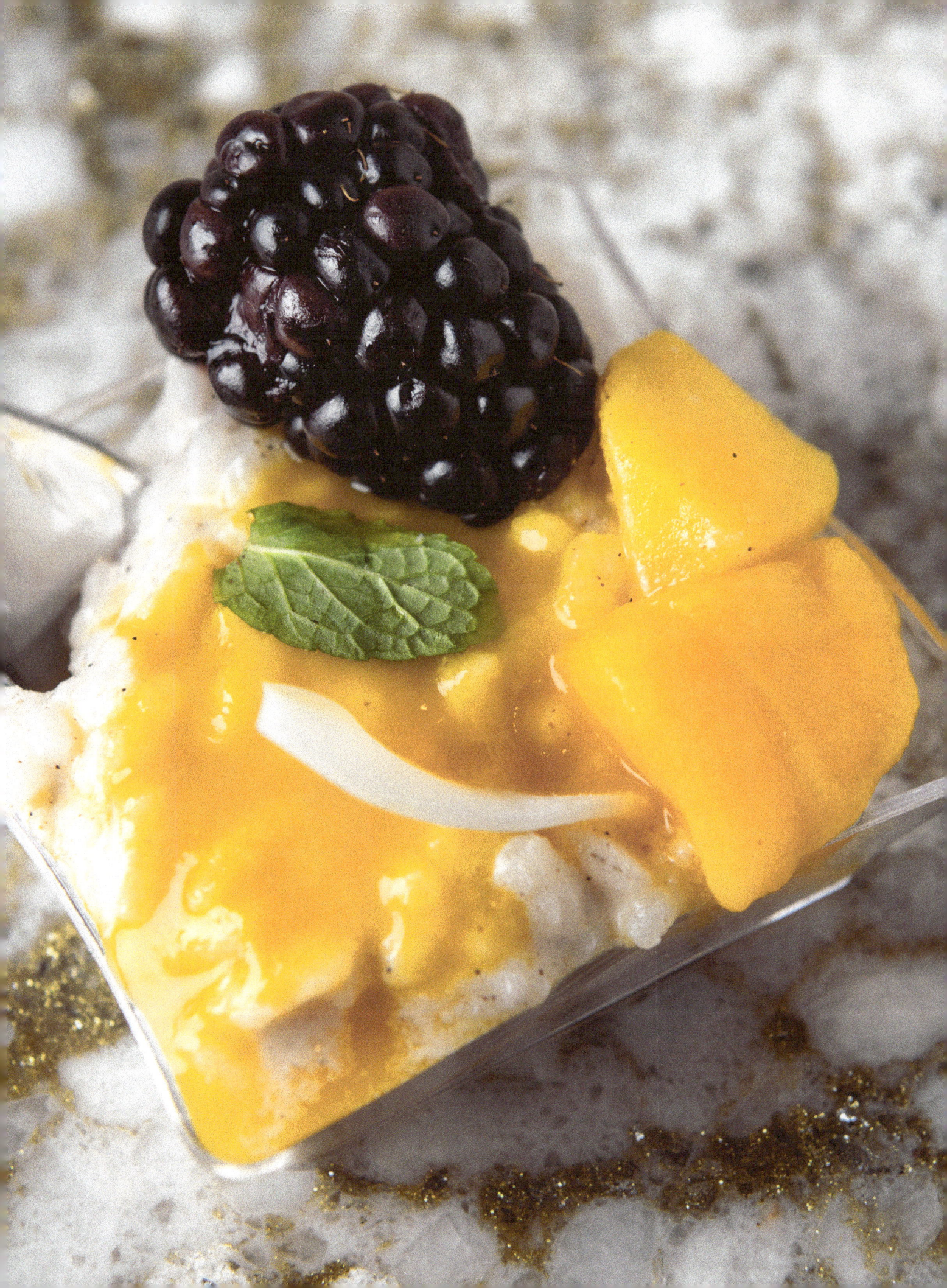

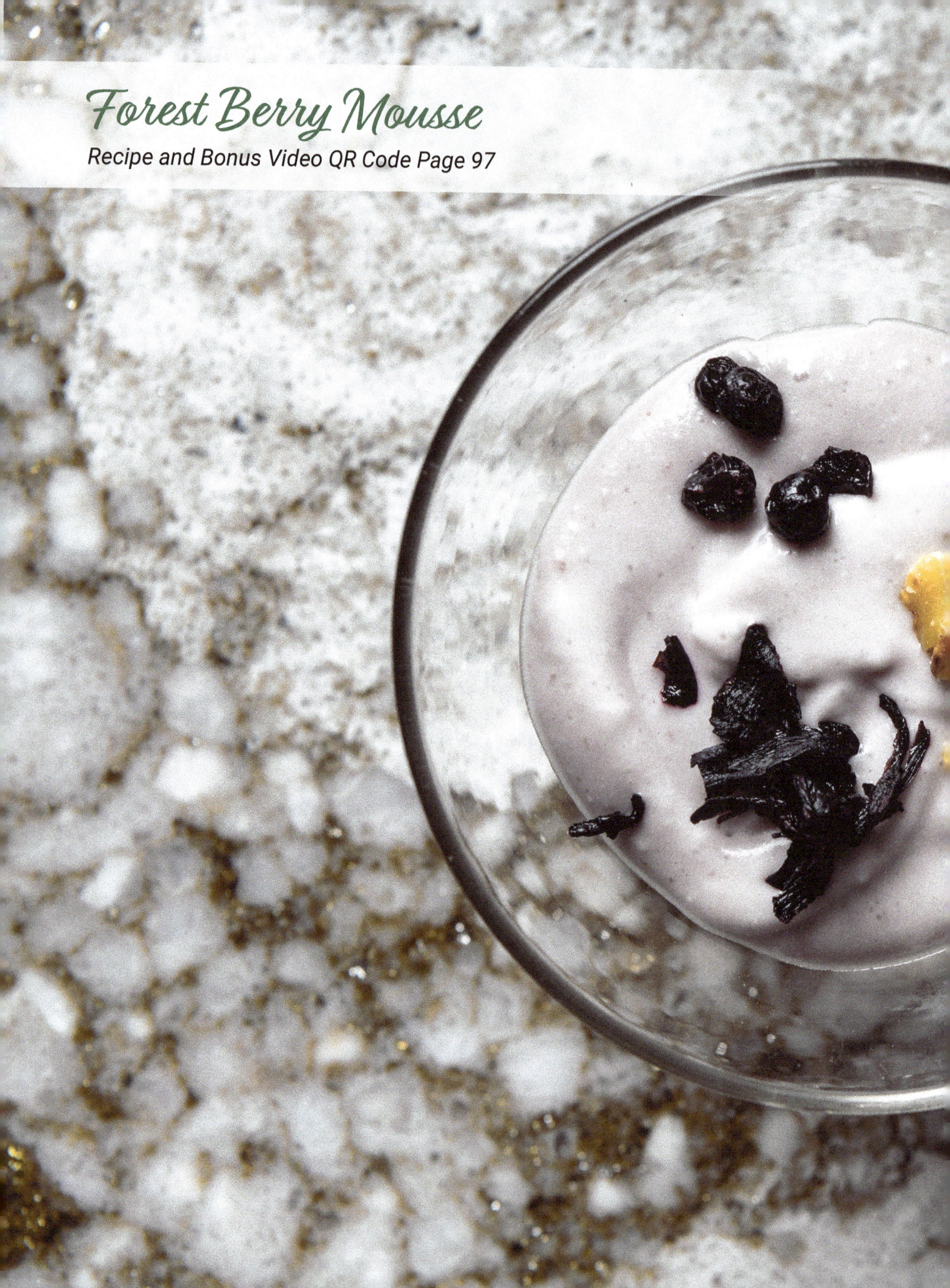

Forest Berry Mousse

Recipe and Bonus Video QR Code Page 97

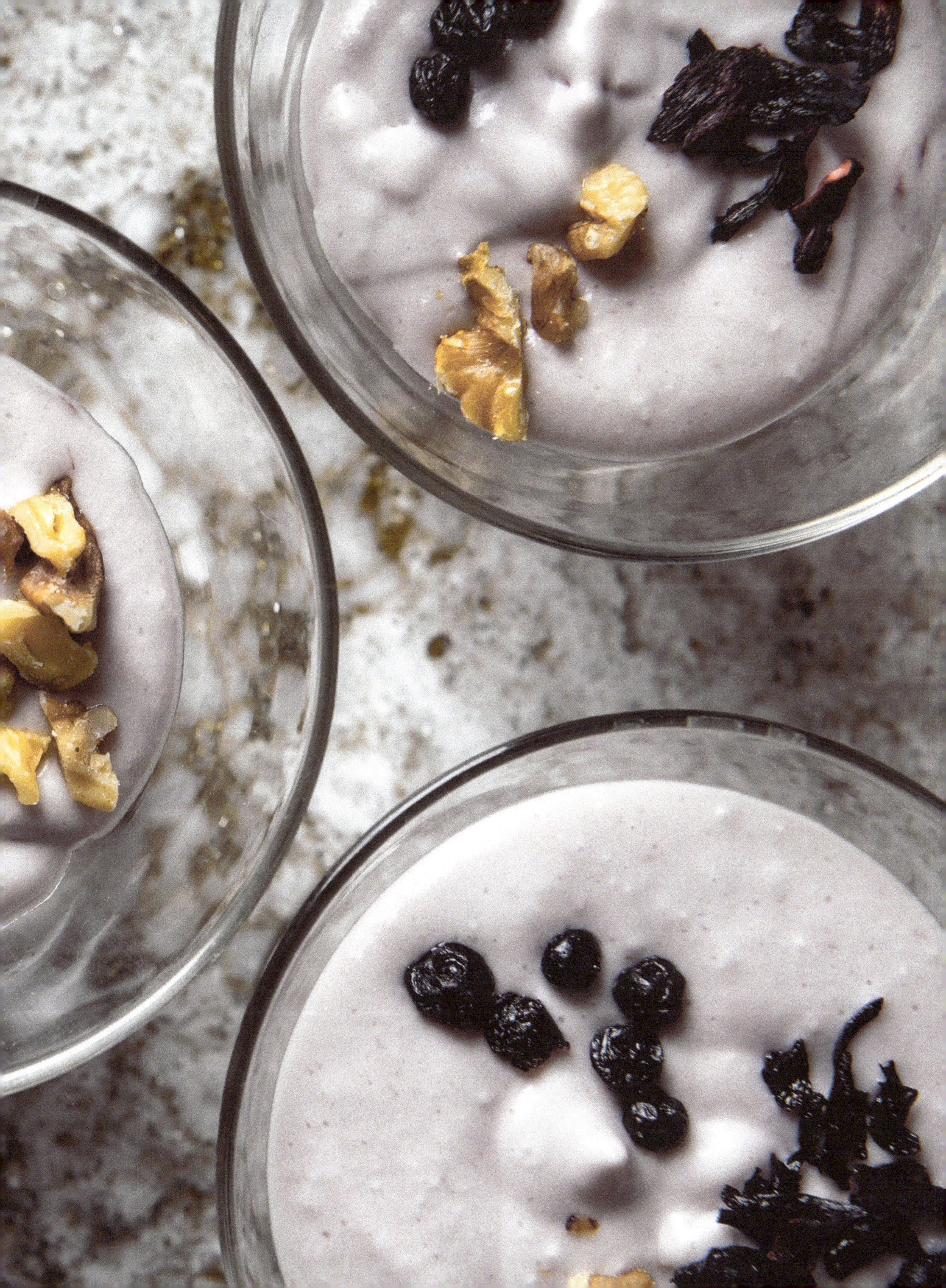

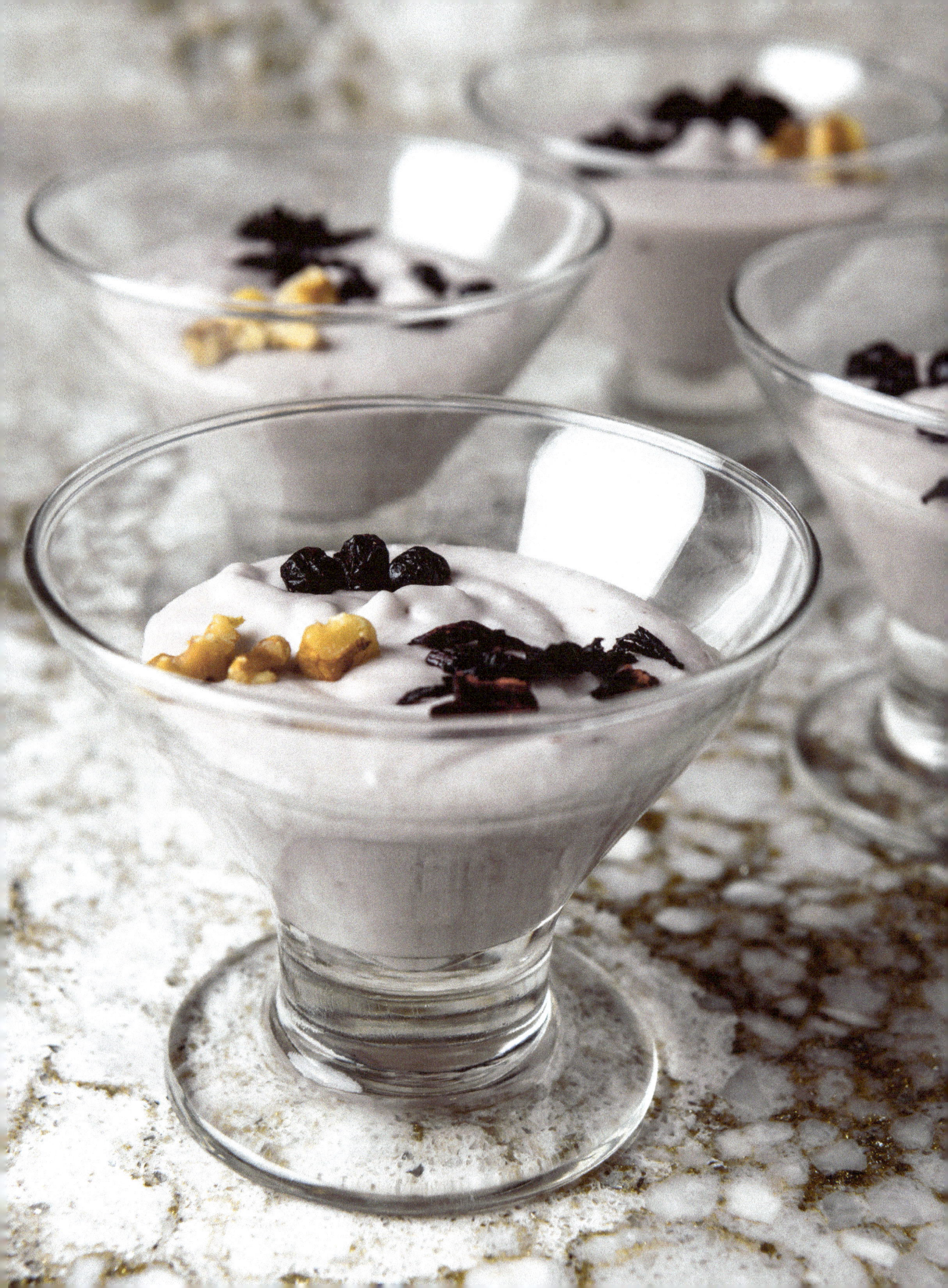

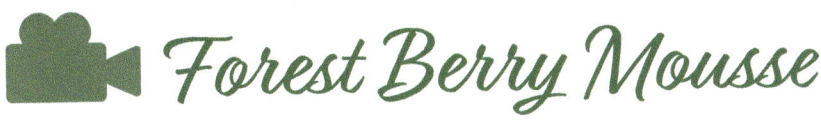

Forest Berry Mousse

Equipment: Large, stainless steel mixing bowl, whisk mixer attachment

2 13 oz. pre-chilled cans of coconut crème with water removed

2 tablespoons of corn starch (organic non-GMO)

1 cup of organic powdered sugar

1 container of Forager Whipped Cream, or any non-dairy whipped cream

⅓ cup of forest berry preserves or any berry preserves

½ teaspoon of Himalayan salt

Optional: 1 tablespoon raspberry liqueur

Garnish:

½ cup of chopped walnuts

¼ cup of dried wild blueberries or candied hibiscus flowers

Directions:

Combine all ingredients, except garnish, in a cold stainless-steel bowl using a whip mixer attachment. Mix at the highest speed for 3 minutes. Refrigerate for a minimum of 2 hours.

With a spatula, scrape all the contents from the mixing bowl into a large Ziploc bag and freeze for at least 1 hour. Thaw for 15 minutes before serving. Slice a corner of the Ziploc and squeeze the mousse into small parfait glasses. You pick the serving size per person. I like about 4 to 6 ounces per person.

Garnish with chopped walnuts and my preference, candied hibiscus flowers.

Serves 6.

Bonus VIDEO TUTORIAL

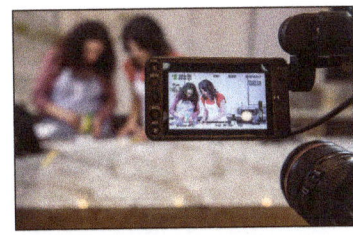

Password: Z1977Fsg1111$
Note: Save the password to your browser for easier access

Raw Pumpkin Power Bites
with White Chocolate Icing

Equipment: Food processor, cookie sheet, small scooper, small microwave-safe mixing bowl

7–8 large Medjool dates, pits removed

3 tablespoons of real maple syrup

1 cup canned organic pumpkin

1½ tablespoons of pumpkin pie spice

2 heaping tablespoons of almond or cashew butter

1 tablespoon of vanilla bean paste

1 packet of Arbonne Vanilla Protein Shake mix, or 1 to 2 scoops of vegan vanilla protein powder of your choice

1 cup of pumpkin granola or granola of choice (gluten-free)

½ cup of hemp seeds or hearts, shelled

1 cup of gluten-free bran flakes

¾ cup of almond meal

1 cup gluten-free all-purpose flour OR 1 cup of oat flour

½ teaspoon of kosher salt

Optional: add ½ cup of pumpkins seeds to the dough

Filling

2 vegan white chocolate almond candy bars

Icing

1 package of rice milk white chocolate chips (Natural Grocers or Vitamin Cottage Store)*

1 tablespoon of coconut oil

½ teaspoon of cinnamon

Directions:

Combine power bite ingredients in a food processor and blend at high speed for at least 3 to 4 minutes. Form the mixture into 1½ tablespoon-sized ball-shaped bites. Lay power bites onto a wax paper-lined cookie sheet and put them in the fridge for a minimum of 1 hour. Meanwhile, break each white chocolate square into four small pieces. Each white chocolate candy bar will yield 16 pieces.

Push each of the white chocolate pieces into a power bite and refrigerate for an additional hour. Next, add rice milk chocolate chips, and cinnamon into a small glass bowl with coconut oil, and microwave at 50% heat for 3 minutes. Remove from microwave and whisk to a liquid consistency. Cool for three minutes. Drizzle the white chocolate with a spoon over each pumpkin bite until all bites are covered in a white chocolate drizzle. Refrigerate for an additional 20 minutes before eating.

This recipe makes 24 servings. They will keep in the fridge for up to one week.

*May be purchased online.

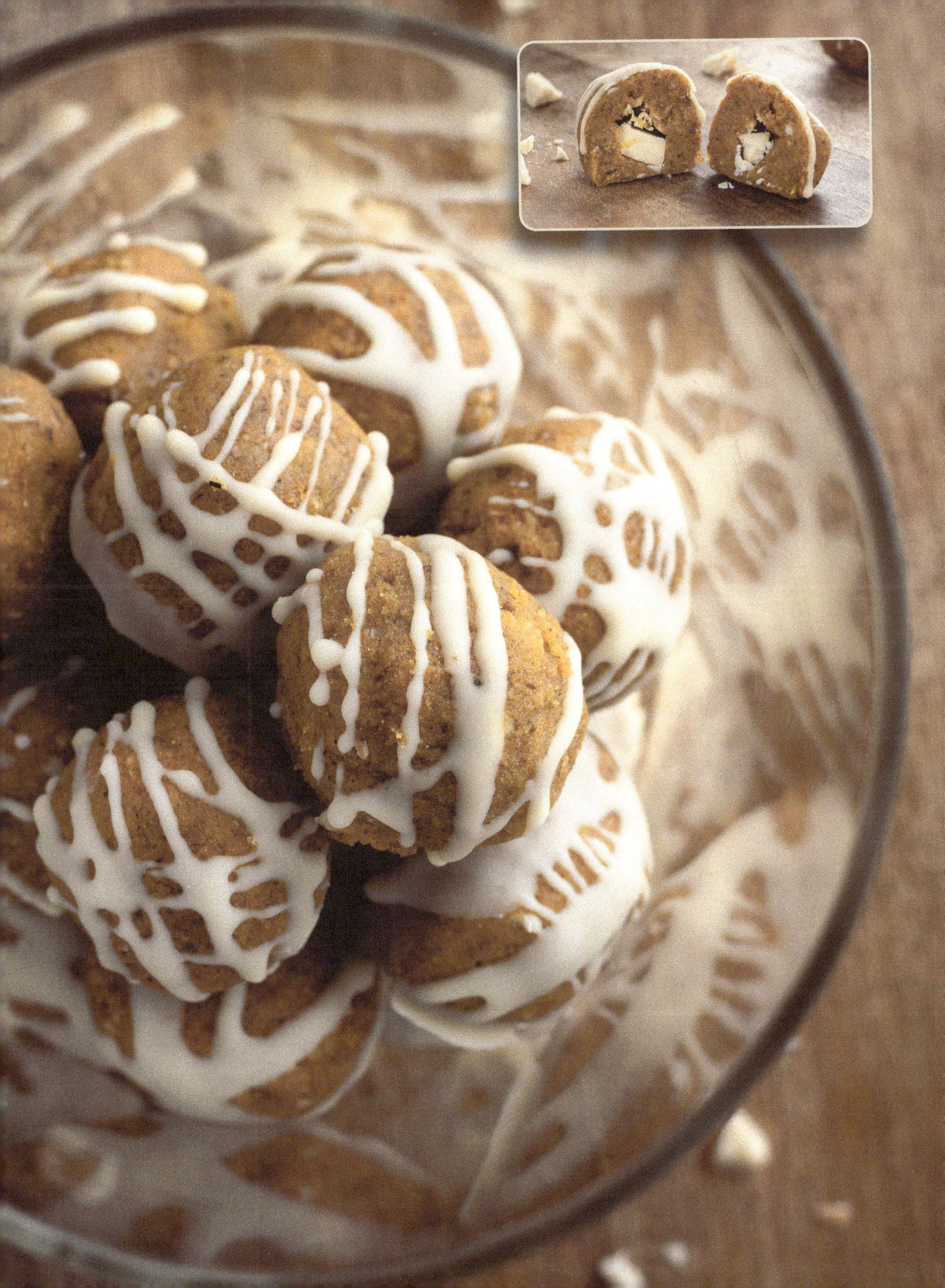

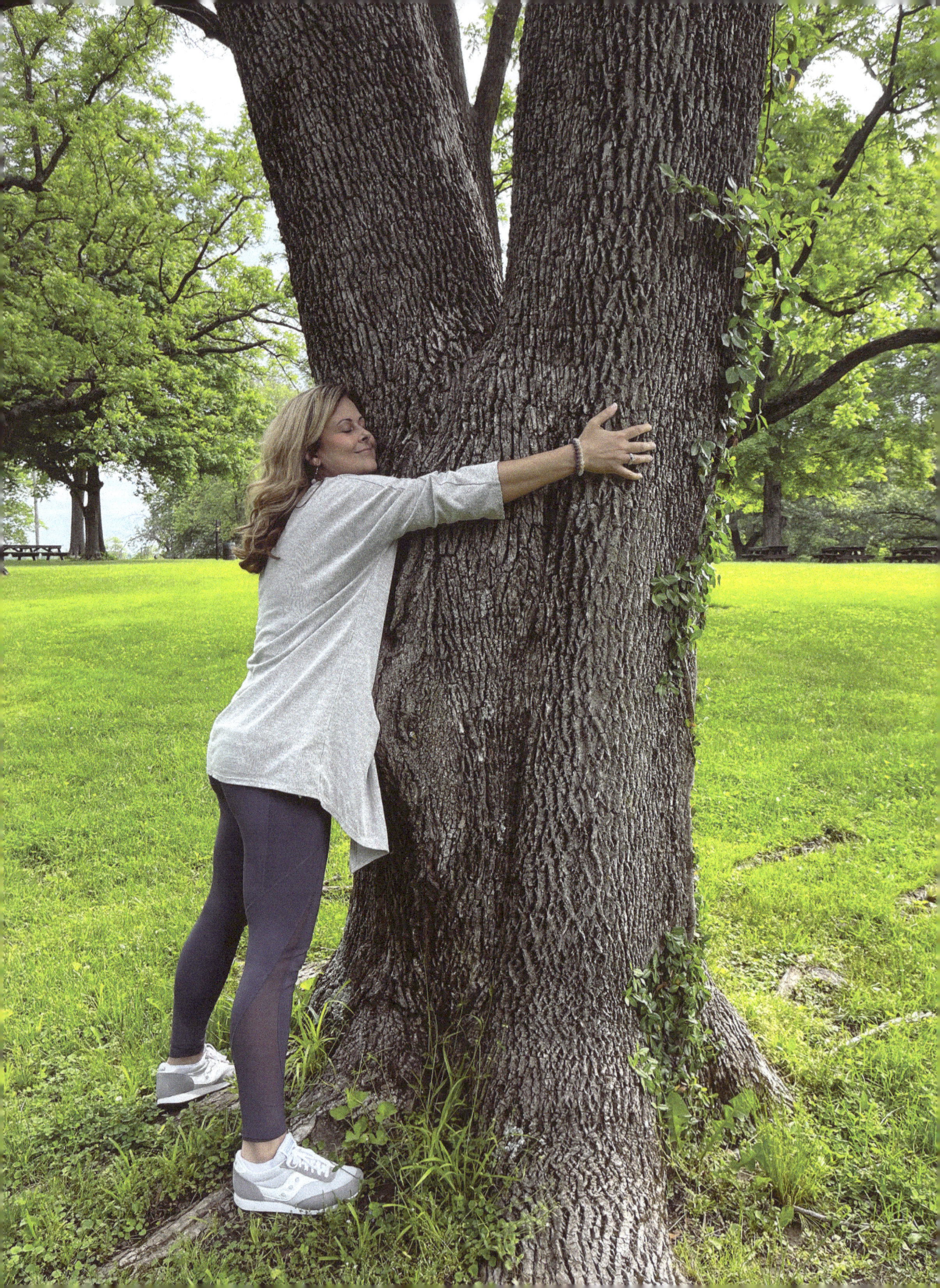

Chef Tips and Tricks

Working as a chef for many years, I've come up with several quick yet effective ways to make food taste better. First, it's about seasoning every layer of the food as you prepare it. When you're sautéing, roasting, or basting your food dishes, season them lightly at least three times with salt and pepper until you get your finished dish completed. Sometimes, you can salt or pepper to your dish once again at the end. Taste, season, taste, season, and repeat.

Other Tips and Tricks

- Blanch veggies like Brussels sprouts, green beans, broccoli, and cabbage first in salted boiled water for 2 to 3 minutes before roasting, sautéing, or frying. It will take the bitterness and sharpness out of these vegetables. It will also caramelize the sweeter flavors in these vegetables and make them more palatable.

- Don't be afraid to combine textures of foods to add more variety and unique flavor to your dishes. For example, I like to add pumpkin seeds for that extra crunch in Mexican dishes. I like to drizzle toasted sesame oil on Asian dishes after they are cooked just like you drizzle extra virgin olive oil on Italian dishes at the end as a finishing garnish. In desserts, I enjoy adding specialty liqueurs to mousses and icings and even cake batter for that special addition not many people can identify but love.

- When I particularly adore a sauce that I created, I make a double batch so that I have plenty to spread around liberally. Have you ever seen a guest or friend lick their plate? I see it all the time. It's the best compliment to the chef. If you give them extra sauce, they usually don't have to go to such extreme measures.

- If you prep a dish ahead of time that has pasta or rice in it, always cook it for 2 to 3 minutes under the time required. So, when you reheat or incorporate those items into your finished dish, they are not overdone. I don't enjoy food that is overdone or mushy, and most people don't.

- Feel free to add food-grade essential oils to salad dressings, icings, sauces, and teas. Here's a quick trick I like to use frequently: take a milk-frothing tool and buzz the essential oil drop into the liquid part of the recipe thoroughly before adding the rest of the ingredients. Essential oils are very potent and the only time they are off-putting is when they are not emulsified properly. This will ensure that there are only hints of the flavor instead of an overly tart or bitter taste.

- Experiment with using date paste, maple syrup, prickly pear syrup, and other fruit and natural sweeteners in your recipes instead of sugar. Most of the time, they provide a much better taste than sugar.

...more tips next page

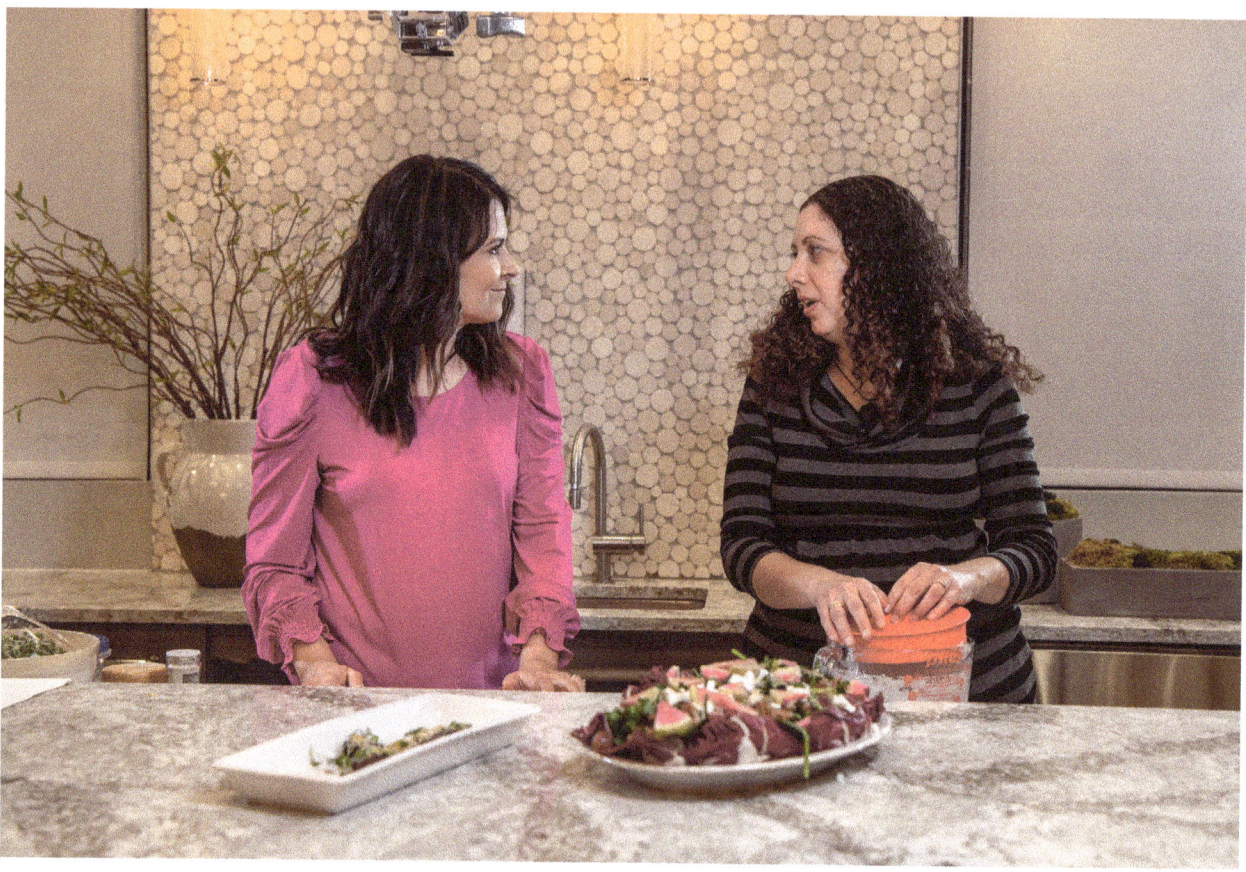

- With vegan cooking, feel free to overuse items like mushroom powder, miso paste, miso broths, and nutritional yeast for that umami flavor that typically only meat, dairy, and eggs can provide.

- Don't be shy about using pickle juice, almond butter, and mustard in your recipes as an extra flavor component. This is a technique used by chefs and resourceful cooks to experiment. When I make "deviled potatoes" (you can find several recipes on Pinterest), I always add a teaspoon of sweet pickle juice to the mixture for that classic taste. If I have extra taco sauce left over, I add it to my Mexican food bowls for that spicy, unusual addition.

- Always find a fresh herb to add to your dish in some way. Fresh herbs add brightness and freshness to dishes that cannot be replicated. If you have a canned ingredient in your recipe, adding a fresh herb will mask that the ingredient is not fresh. Also, adding fresh lemon or lime juice to most dishes lifts that fresh taste.

- Take your vegetable food scraps and make a homemade broth. Add water and bay leaves and you have a broth after simmering on low for a couple of hours.

- Cook or roast not-so-pretty vegetable scraps and add them to rice or noodle bowls. Nine times out of ten, adding more vegetables makes the dish taste more amazing.

Chef Tips and Tricks

- If a recipe doesn't call for a particular ingredient, but you think it would taste good, add it anyway. The worst thing that will happen is that you won't be doing it again. However, most of the time I love adding weird vegetables or ingredients that the recipe didn't call for; it always adds an unusual yet great taste to the modified dish.

- Edible flowers are so pretty on the plate! Add them whenever you want a fancy, perfect garnish.

- Make a hash out of vegetable scraps in the morning for breakfast. Combine as many as you want along with potatoes. Pile them on top of each other and drizzle with your favorite sauce. Using leftovers means no waste and can make for a great meal.

- For white sauces like alfredo, use pea protein plant milk instead of any other plant milk. It does not give an aftertaste like other plant milks after cooking.

- Do not freeze avocados. They do not taste good after thawing, and neither do asparagus and celery. Some items taste horrible no matter how you cook them after thawing, and they shouldn't be frozen in the first place.

- After you finish preparing a dish, stand back and look at its colors. Can a green, pink, orange, red, or purple garnish be added for color? Can a white creamy sauce be a pretty base for darker food? Can a drizzle of oil add a silky green look to a darker sauce? So many items can be added to your dish for color. After all, we eat with our eyes.

- If you think you didn't make enough food for a group, serve bread, crackers, and dip or fun little appetizers like the ones I've shared in this book before the main course. Make them pretty and conversational, announcing what each snack consists of in detail.

Chef Frances' Famous Feta Cheeseballs
Recipe Page 27

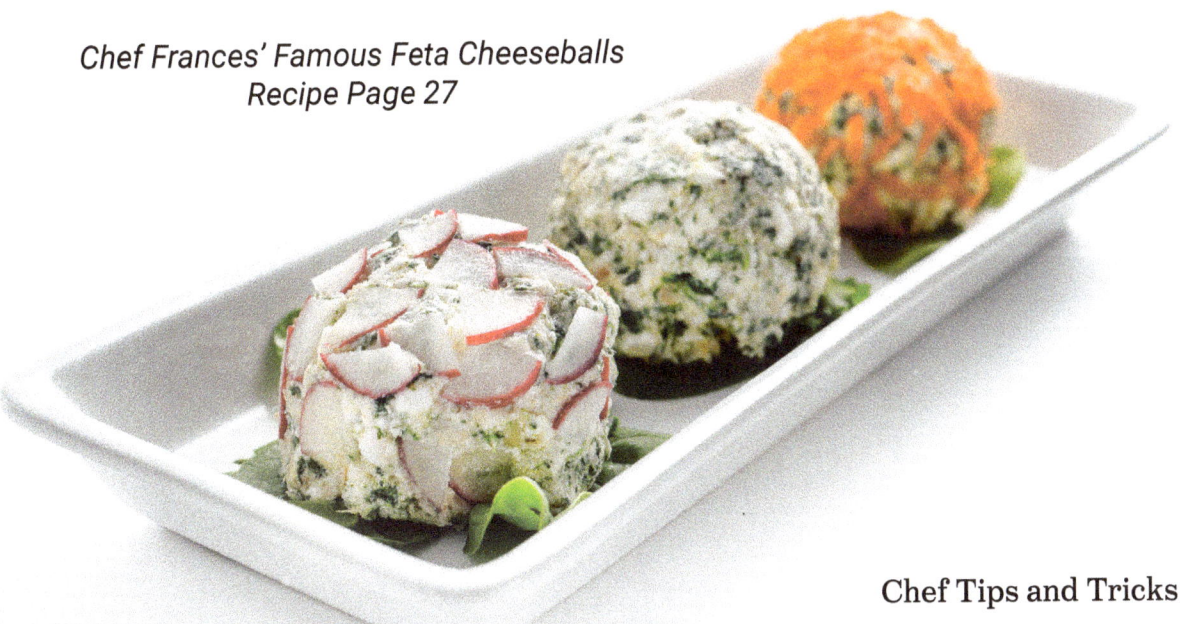

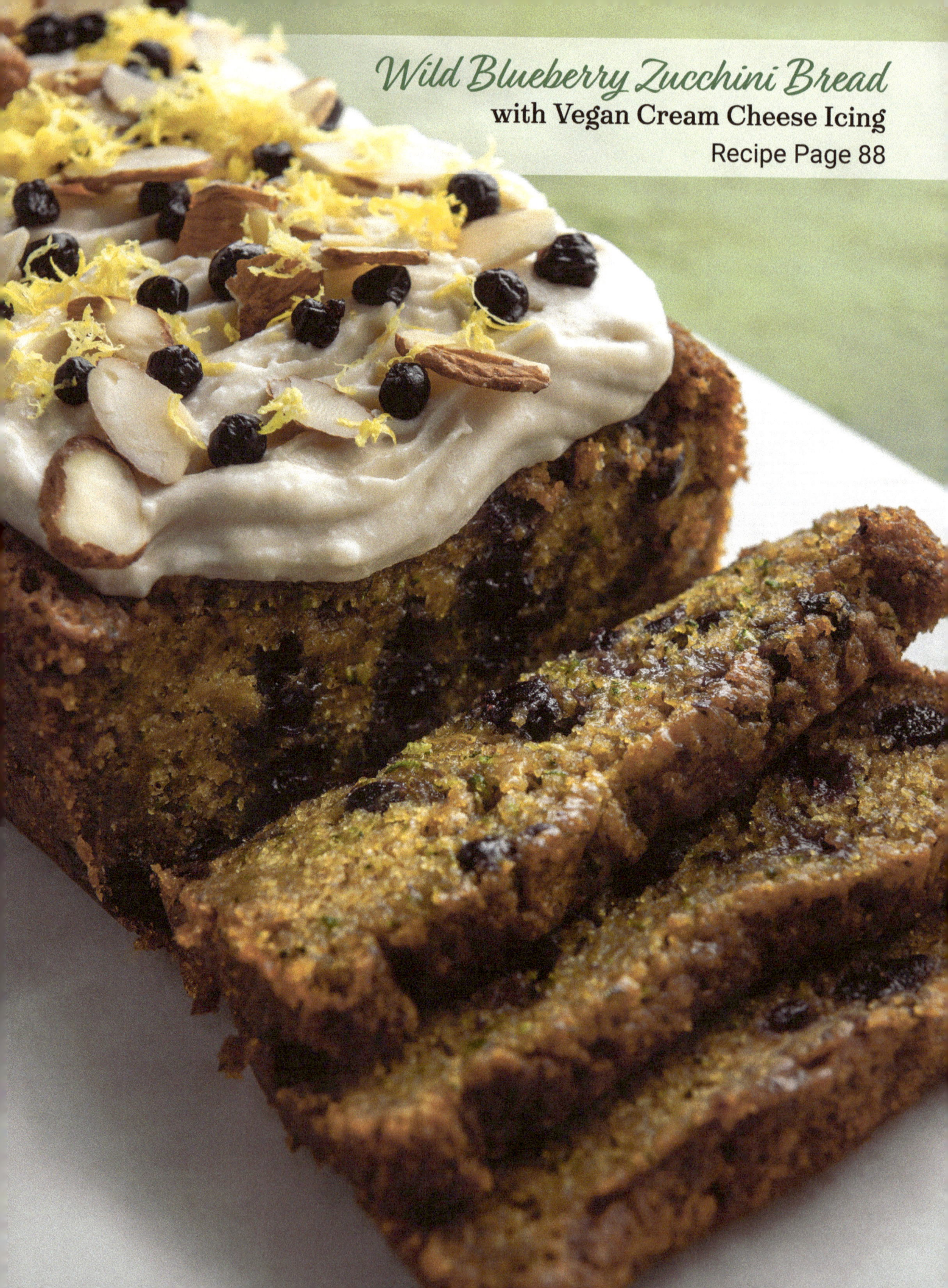

Wild Blueberry Zucchini Bread
with Vegan Cream Cheese Icing
Recipe Page 88

Index

Coconut Crème
    Midwest-Style Vegan Corn Chowder, *25*
    Coconut Crème Balsamic Dressing, *49*
    Vegan Bread Pudding, *91*
    Forest Berry Mousse, *97*
Coconut Milk
    Sticky Rice Pudding with Mango Purée and Coconut Chips, *92*
Corn, Corn Chips, Corn Tortilla
    Midwest-Style Corn Chowder, *25*
    Pineapple and Avocado Salad, *42*
    Carne Asada Potato Enchiladas, *70*
    Crispy, Sweet Corn Griddle Cakes, *74*
Cream Cheese
    Chef Frances' Famous Feta Cheeseballs, *27*
    Vegan Cream Cheese Icing, *89*
Croissants
    Vegan Bread Pudding, *91*
Daring Plant Chicken Tenders
    Veggie and Daring Chicken Skewers, *56*
Dates
    Raw Pumpkin Power Bites with White Chocolate Icing, *98*
Edamame
    Sweet Potato Bowl with High-protein Pink Dressing, *40*
Feta
    Chef Frances' Famous Feta Cheeseballs, *27*
    Grape Quinoa Salad with a Coconut Crème, Balsamic Dressing, *49*
Flaxseed
    Crispy, Sweet Corn Griddle Cakes, *74*
    Wild Blueberry Zucchini Bread with Vegan Cream Cheese Icing, *88*
Gardein Beefless Tips
    Steak and Yukon Gold Potato Bites, *83*
Gluten-free Bran Flakes
    Raw Pumpkin Power Bites with White Chocolate Icing, *98*
Granola
    Raw Pumpkin Power Bites with White Chocolate Icing, *98*
Hearts of Palm
    Vegan Crab Cakes, *61*
Hemp, Seeds, Hearts
    Raw Pumpkin Power Bites with White Chocolate Icing, *98*
Ian's Original Panko, Gluten-free Breadcrumbs
    Stuffed Mushrooms with Microgreens, *31*
    Cold Angel Hair Pasta with Roma Tomatoes and Aromatic Italian Dressing, *46*
    Vegan Crab Cakes, *61*
    Vegan Shepherd's Pie, *66*

Shallots
  Midwest-Style Vegan Corn Chowder, *25*
  Cauliflower Power Side Salad, *45*
  Israeli Couscous and Kale Salad, *50*
  Vegan Beurre Blanc, *54*
  Mushroom Risotto with Roasted Red Peppers and Sweet Peas, *59*
  Vegan Shepherd's Pie, *66*
  Crispy, Sweet Corn Griddle Cakes, *74*
Spinach
  Chef Frances' Famous Feta Cheeseballs, *27*
  Caesar Pasta Salad with Baby Kale, Chard and Spinach, *37*
  Grape Quinoa Salad, *49*
  Tomato and Spinach JUST Egg Omelet, *62*
Sweet Peas
  Mushroom Risotto with Roasted Red Peppers and Sweet Peas Sweet Peas, *59*
Sweet Potato
  Sweet Potato Bowl, *40*
  Breakfast Hash, *58*
Sweet Potato Flour
  Crispy, Sweet Corn Griddle Cakes, *74*
Tomato, Roma
  Cold Angel Hair Pasta with Roma Tomatoes, *46*
  Tomato and Spinach JUST Egg Omelet, *62*
Tortillas
  Pineapple and Avocado Salad, *42*
  Carne Asada Potato Enchiladas, *70*
Unbleached Cane Sugar
  Creamy Pomegranate Dressing, *42*
  Homemade Enchilada Sauce, *70*
  Wild Blueberry Zucchini Bread, *88*
  Sticky Rice Pudding with Mango Purée and Coconut Chips, *92*
Vanilla, Bean Paste, Extract
  Wild Blueberry Zucchini Bread, *88*
  Vegan Bread Pudding, *91*
  Raw Pumpkin Power Bites with White Chocolate Icing, *98*
Vegan Mayo
  Chef Frances' Famous Feta Cheeseballs, *27*
  Cashew Caesar Dressing, *37*
  Creamy Pomegranate Dressing, *42*
  Agave Mustard Dressing, *45*
  Steak and Yukon Gold Potato Bites, *83*

Pesto Potato Poppers, *84*

Vegetable Broth
- French Onion Soup, *33*
- Midwest-Style Vegan Corn Chowder, *25*
- Grape Quinoa Salad, *49*
- Mushroom Risotto with Roasted Red Peppers and Sweet Peas, *59*
- Vegan Shepherd's Pie, *66*
- Miso Mashed Potatoes, *79*

Vinegar, Balsamic, Champagne, Apple Cider, Red Wine, White Wine
- Cashew Caesar Dressing, *37*
- High-Protein Pink Dressing, *41*
- Creamy Pomegranate Dressing, *42*
- Agave Mustard Dressing, *45*
- Aromatic Italian Dressing, *46*
- Coconut Crème Balsamic Dressing, *49*
- Mouthwatering Vinaigrette Recipe, *50*
- Sweet and Tangy Dressing, *51*

Violife Cheese
- Chef Frances' Famous Feta Cheeseballs, *27*
- French Onion Soup, *33*
- Grape Quinoa Salad, *49*
- Tomato and Spinach JUST Egg Omelet, *62*

Walnuts
- Stuffed Poblano Peppers, *74*
- Forest Berry Mousse, *97*

Worcestershire Sauce
- French Onion Soup, *33*
- Veggie and Daring Chicken Skewers, *56*
- Vegan Shepherd's Pie, *66*
- Steak and Yukon Gold Potato Bites, *83*

Zucchini
- Sweet Potato Bowl with High-Protein Pink Dressing, *40*
- Veggie and Daring Chicken Skewers, *56*
- Breakfast Hash, *58*
- Carne Asada Potato Enchiladas, *70*
- Calabacitas, *74*
- Wild Blueberry Zucchini Bread with Vegan Cream Cheese Icing, *88*

About the Author

Frances Star Graham is a private vegan chef, plant-based educator, quantum sound healer, and qigong instructor. From 2009 to 2014—from the ages of 32 to 37, she was bedridden three months per year and struggled with chronic pain and fatigue related to four serious autoimmune diseases: Sjögren's, Hashimoto, Scleroderma, and Raynaud's Syndrome.

In 2013, Frances had a near-death experience while going through a routine medical procedure. After this fight or flight situation, she went searching for ways to heal herself. This journey began through practicing qigong, tai chi, meridian stretching, tapping, and other healing modalities. After a year, she was able to regenerate her thyroid gland to normal size after losing 40% of the entire gland due to Hashimoto's disease. Two years later, after converting to a plant-based diet along with regular qigong classes, Frances was in remission with only mild symptoms, and she was no longer bedridden or experiencing chronic fatigue. Currently, Frances teaches weekly qigong classes and has a thriving career as a private vegan chef and quantum sound healer.

Frances lives with her husband of 21 years and son who is in his second year of college. She has one daughter who lives in Arizona and is an amazing cook. She is originally from Springfield, Illinois, and she enjoys taking her homestyle way of eating from the Midwest and transforming those dishes into vegan comfort food. She currently loves to hike and travel the world in her spare time.

Supporting others on their journey through self-healing is her life mission.

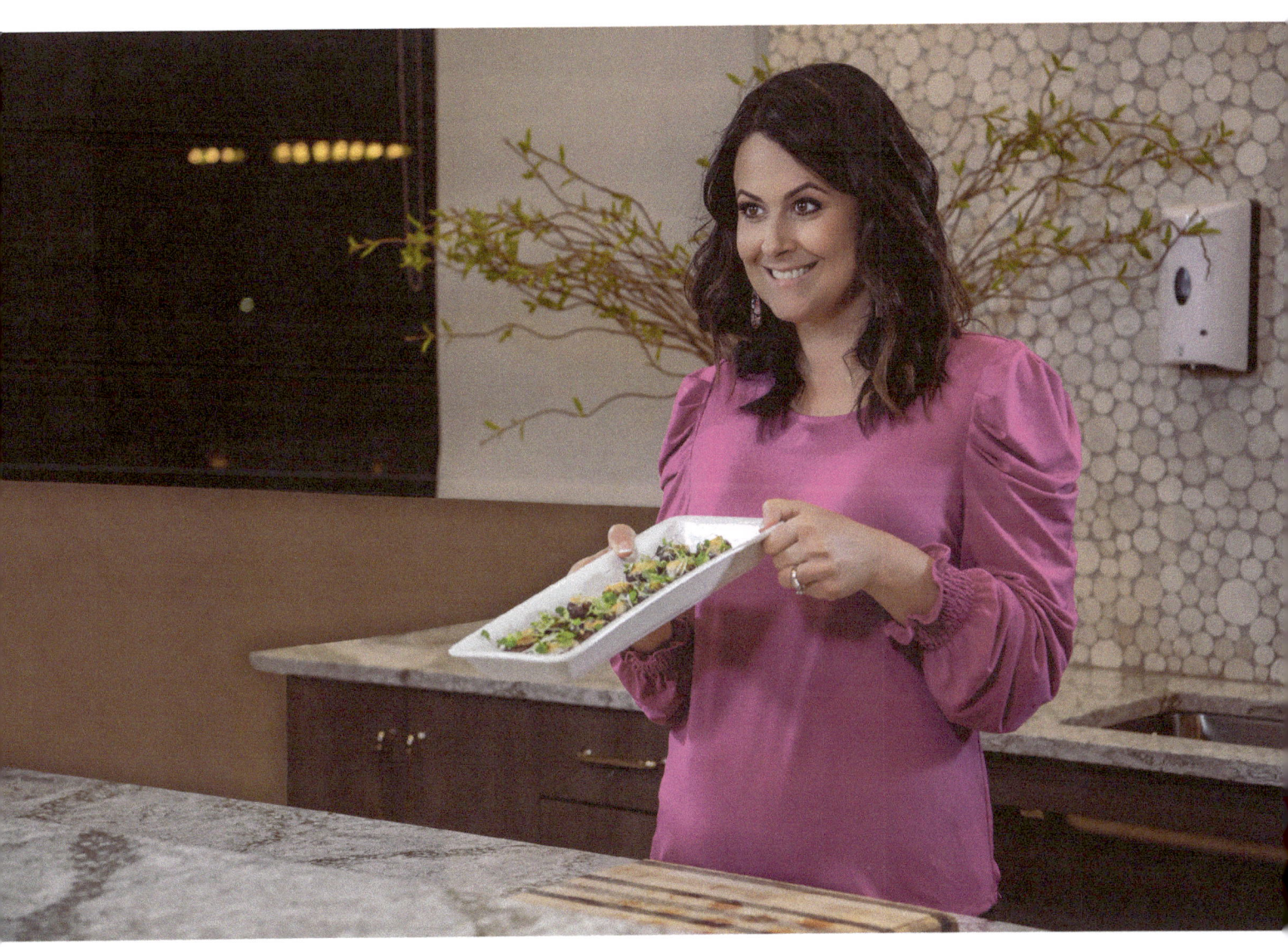